Introduction to General Pharmacy

Second Edition

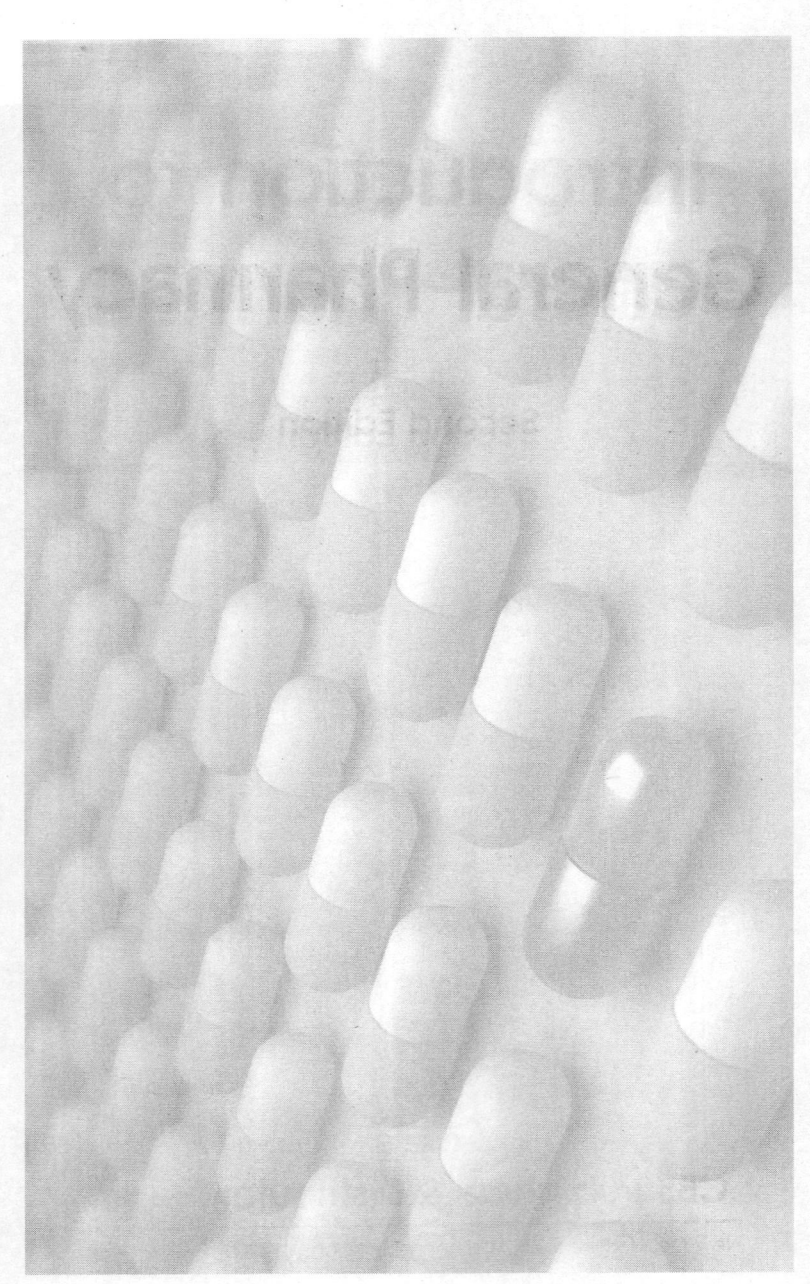

Introduction to General Pharmacy

Second Edition

Gaurav Agarwal

MPharm (BITS-Pilani) PhD

Dean
Faculty of Pharmacy
RP Educational Trust
Karnal, Haryana

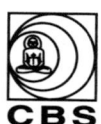

CBS

CBS Publishers & Distributors Pvt Ltd

New Delhi • Bengaluru • Chennai • Kochi • Kolkata • Mumbai
Hyderabad • Nagpur • Patna • Pune • Vijayawada

Introduction to General Pharmacy

Second Edition

ISBN: 978-81-239-2929-3

Copyright © Author and Publisher

Second Edition: 2016

First Edition: 2014

Published by Satish Kumar Jain and produced by Varun Jain for

CBS Publishers & Distributors Pvt Ltd

4819/XI Prahlad Street, 24 Ansari Road, Daryaganj, New Delhi 110 002, India.

Ph: 23289259, 23266861, 23266867   Website: www.cbspd.com

Fax: 011-23243014   e-mail: delhi@cbspd.com; cbspubs@airtelmail.in.

Corporate Office: 204 FIE, Industrial Area, Patparganj, Delhi 110 092

Ph: 4934 4934   Fax: 4934 4935   e-mail: publishing@cbspd.com; publicity@cbspd.com

Branches

- **Bengaluru:** Seema House 2975, 17th Cross, K.R. Road,
  Banasankari 2nd Stage, Bengaluru 560 070, Karnataka
  Ph: +91-80-26771678/79   Fax: +91-80-26771680   e-mail: bangalore@cbspd.com
- **Chennai:** 7, Subbaraya Street, Shenoy Nagar, Chennai 600 030, Tamil Nadu
  Ph: +91-44-26680620, 26681266   Fax: +91-44-42032115   e-mail: chennai@cbspd.com
- **Kochi:** Ashana House, No. 39/1904, AM Thomas Road, Valanjambalam,
  Ernakulam 682 018, Kochi, Kerala
  Ph: +91-484-4059061-65   Fax: +91-484-4059065   e-mail: kochi@cbspd.com
- **Kolkata:** 6/B, Ground Floor, Rameswar Shaw Road, Kolkata-700 014, West Bengal
  Ph: +91-33-22891126, 22891127, 22891128   e-mail: kolkata@cbspd.com
- **Mumbai:** 83-C, Dr E Moses Road, Worli, Mumbai-400018, Maharashtra
  Ph: +91-22-24902340/41   Fax: +91-22-24902342   e-mail: mumbai@cbspd.com

Representatives

- **Hyderabad** 0-9885175004   • **Nagpur** 0-9021734563   • **Patna** 0-9334159340
- **Pune** 0-9623451994   • **Vijayawada** 0-9000660880

Printed at : Swastik Packagings, 506 F.I.E. Patparganj, Delhi - 92

to
my loving kids
Shreya and Vaidish

Foreword

It is our privilege to write a few words about Dr Gaurav Agarwal's second edition *Introduction to General Pharmacy*. This book is a ready-reckoner for B Pharmacy students.

Efforts have been mainly made to focus on the primary aspects for students of pharmacy undergoing degree and diploma courses of various degree/diploma awarding bodies. It seems to be one of the finest efforts of its own kind to offer a wide range of various fundamentals in the field of pharmaceutics from the very traditional to the modern trends of sciences and cutting-edge technologies of today. Pharmaceutics being an interdisciplinary subject, today covering a wide range of interest both among the students and teaching communities. We compliment the author for simple and explicit presentation. And sure that this book is going to become popular and sought after by pharmacy students. We wish the author success in his present venture and urge him to continue this good and noble work by publishing more books for the benefit of pharmacy students.

Dr Agarwal is to be congratulated for the tremendous efforts he has made in compiling this useful work for budding pharmacy technocrats. The present book admirably fills up various gaps between the pharmacy students and the basic knowledge required for specialized training of the subject. He has distilled his vast experience of teaching and research for pharmacy students in this compact and concise text for students and teachers of pharmacy.

Presently Dr Agarwal is working with RPIIT, an institution of par excellence which has reached unflinching success in its strides for imparting quality education. As it is the largest integrated, Hi-tech, state-of-art facilitated private campus in Northern India located at Karnal (Haryana), RPIIT institute is presently offering various technical and professional courses like B Tech, B Arch, B Pharmacy, MBA, PGDBM affiliated to

Kurukshetra University, and BPT, Nursing and BASLP courses affiliated to Pt BD Sharma University of Health Sciences, Rohtak (Haryana), India. The main objective of the institute is to train the students in such a manner that they can consider every problem as a challenge, transform every challenge into opportunity, seize every opportunity and ensure growth in every aspect of life by utilizing all the technical skills imbibed.

Dr Rajiv Singal
Vice Chairman
RP Educational Trust
Karnal, Haryana

Dr Nidhi Singal
Managing Director
RP Educational Trust
Karnal, Haryana

Preface to the Second Edition

The book *Introduction to General Pharmacy* has been well received both by the academician and the students undergoing diploma and degree in pharmacy as its first edition. The revised and updated second edition contains valuable additions in chapters on prescription, incompatibility in prescriptions and lot of new experiments in pharmaceutics. This edition of the book is a result of an initiative to keep abreast of the timely and critical changing roles and responsibilities of pharmaceutics. It has been my pleasure to edit and maintain the objective of previous edition. The book has been so well received by the readers and also the feedback they have provided. We hope this edition will further ameliorate the conceptual approach towards the understanding of pharmaceutics.

Revision has been made in almost all the chapters to include more diagrams and examples so as to make the subject easily understandable.

I am grateful to my readers, especially the faculty members for their critical comments. I am thankful to Mr YN Arjuna of CBSPD and his team for providing continuous support and patience during the revision of this edition.

In spite of a great care, there might be some mistakes and deficiencies. I will be grateful for giving suggestions to improve upon myself. I appreciate the readers to point out those deficiencies and do mail to me at *gbitsian@rediffmail.com*. The constructive suggestions for improvement are always welcome.

Gaurav Agarwal

Preface to the First Edition

This book *Introduction to General Pharmacy* is expected to be one of its kind to span a wide gamut of basic pharmaceutics from the very traditional to what is cutting edge today. This book although designated for entry-level students, covers wide areas. It contains a comprehensive description an overview of existing knowledge of pharmaceutics and making it appropriate for introductory and institutional purposes.

Being an interdisciplinary subject, it is today covering a wide range of interest both among the students and teaching communities. Taking this increasing interest into account, this book gives a comprehensives introduction to the subject. The text not only deals with the basic concepts but also emphasizes technical and practical aspects of the subject. The book is primarily intended as text for students of pharmacy for degree and diploma courses.

The book contains numerous specimens, vivid illustrations, tables, diagrams and flow diagrams to present the ideas. The distinguishing feature is ample question bank at the end of the book. In spite of great care there might be some mistakes and deficiencies. I will be grateful for giving suggestions to improve upon myself. So go through the content and do mail to me at *gbitsian@rediffmail.com*. Because you share that spirit, the book is dedicated to you.

Gaurav Agarwal

Acknowledgments

It is a moment of great pleasure and immense satisfaction for me to express deep gratitude and gratefulness to Prof (Dr) Gajendra Singh, Dean, Faculty of Pharmaceutical Sciences, Pt BD Sharma University of Health Sciences, Rohtak, for inspiring me to bring out this book.

I am specially thankful to Shri RP Singal Ji, Chairman, RP Educational Trust, for his all time support and encouragement.

My special thanks to Er Bharat Singal, Secretary, RP Educational Trust, for inspiring us to bring out this book.

I am indebted to Dr GS Sharma (Director General), Dr Saurabh Gupta (Director), and Dr PK Karar (Principal), Faculty of Pharmacy, RPIIT Technical and Medical Campus, for their motivation.

Special thanks to my peers Ish, Nitesh, Mani, Dr Manish, Manish Kaushik, Jasvinder, Umesh Manju and Satyender for their moral support.

I express my gratefulness to Mr Satish K Jain, CMD, and Mr YN Arjuna, Senior Vice-President, CBS Publishers & Distributors, for their sincere efforts in publishing this book.

Last but not the least, I express my love to my wife Dr Shilpi Agarwal for her all time inspiration and dedication. She is the major driving force in bringing out this achievement.

To our numerous students, whom I cannot possibly name individually, I thanks for their class interactions which have been the guiding spirit in selection of the subject matter and its logical arrangement.

Gaurav Agarwal

Contents

1

History of Pharmacy and Pharmacopoeia

ORIGIN AND DEVELOPMENT OF PHARMACY

'**Bheshaj**' is the term used in India from the last four thousand years which is equivalent to Greek term '**Pharmacon**' meaning drug from which the term Pharmacy has been derived. In ancient times Pharmacist was responsible for making the drug into suitable dosage form acceptable to patient. Pharmacist was also involved in procurement of drug from various sources. Hence, pharmacy is the branch that deals with identification, procurement, formulation and dispensing of drug. In ancient times there was a believe that peoples associated with this profession have some spiritual powers and hence the profession is treated in a different manner by the society. Throughout history, many individual have contributed to the advancement of the health sciences. Notable among those whose genius and creativeness had a revolutionary influence on the development of pharmacy and medicine were **Hippocrates** (ca. 460–377 BC), **Dioscorides** (1st Century AD), **Galen** (ca. 130–200 AD), and **Paracelsus** (1793–1541 AD).

Hippocrates, a Greek physician, is recognized for the introduction of scientific pharmacy and medicine. He streamlined medicine, systematized medical knowledge and put the practice of medicine on a high ethical place. His thinking on the ethics and sciences medicine dominated the medical writings of his and successive generations. His works included the descriptions of hundreds of drugs, and it was during this period that the term 'Pharmakon' came into existence which means a purifying remedy for good only, excel the previous association of a charm or drug for good or for evil purposes,

Because of his revolutionary work in medical science and his motivation teachings and advanced philosophies that have become a part of modern medicine, Hippocrates is called the **Father of Medicine.**

Dioscorides, a Greek physician and botanist, was the first to used botany as an applied science of pharmacy. His work, *De Materia Medica,* is considered a landmark in the development of pharmaceutical botany and in the study of naturally occurring medicinal materials. This area of study is today known as pharmacognosy, a term fomed from two Greek words, "pharmakon" meaning drug and "gnosis" means knowledge. Some of the drugs Dioscorides described, including opium, ergot, and hyoscyamus, continue to have use in medicine. His descriptions of the art of identifying and collecting natural drug products, the methods of their proper storage, and the means of detecting adulterants or contaminants were the standards of that period, established the need for additional work, and set guidelines for future investigators.

Claudius Galen, a Greek pharmacist-physician, created a perfect system of physiology, pathology, and treatment. Galen prepared doctrines that were followed for 1500 years. He was one of the greatest author of his time, he has created 500 treatise on medicine and around 250 treatise on philosophy, law and grammar. His medical writings include descriptions of numerous drugs of natural origin with a large amount of drug formulas and methods of compounding. He originated so many preparations of vegetable drugs by mixing or melting the individual ingredients that the field of pharmaceutical preparations was commonly referred to as "Galenic pharmacy" at that time.

Pharmacy always remained associated with medicine, Pharmacy was officially separated from medicine for the first time in 1240 AD, when a declaration of **Emperor Frederick II** of Germany regulated the practice of pharmacy within the part of his kingdom called the two Sicilies. His announcement separating the two professions acknowledged that pharmacy required special knowledge, skill, initiative, and responsibility. Pharmacists were obligated by oath to prepare reliable drugs of uniform quality according to their art. Any exploitation of the patient through business relations between the pharmacist and the physician was strictly prohibited.

Perhaps no person in history exercised such a revolutionary influence on pharmacy and medicine as did **Aureolus Theophrastus Bombastus von Hohenheim** (1493–1541), a Swiss physician and chemist who called himself **Paracelsus**. He was the first person who changes the pharmacy from a profession based primarily on botanical science to the one based on chemical science. Some of his chemical observations were astonishing for his time and they become landmark for further discoveries. He emphasize that it was possible to prepare a specific medicinal agent to combat each specific disease and introduced a host of chemical substances to internal therapy. Then further contribution was made by number of scientist by developing new drugs from different sources. In India, the ayurvedic medicine were used as per the ancient books written by **Charak**, a physician, which nowadays replaced by allopathic medicine during the British rule. After independence a new revolutionary era of allopathic medicine leads to further development in pharmaceutical industry. Every person engage with profession of pharmacy has to abide with the pharmacy oath laid down below.

OATH OF A PHARMACIST

At this time, I vow to devote my professional life to the service of all humankind through the profession of pharmacy.

I will consider the welfare of humanity and relief of human suffering, my primary concerns.

I will apply my knowledge, experience, and skills to the best of my ability to assure optimal drug therapy outcomes for the patients I serve.

I will keep abreast of developments and maintain professional competency in my profession of pharmacy. I will maintain the highest principles of moral, ethical and legal conduct.

I will embrace and advocate change in the profession of pharmacy that improves patient care.

I take these vows voluntarily with the full realization of the responsibility with which I am entrusted by the public.

SCOPE OF PHARMACY

From ancient times pharmacy is known as a branch associated with health care services. The word Pharmacy has been derived from the Greek word "Pharmakon", meaning drug. Today, the discipline of pharmacy has made enormous progress and has matured as a distinctly independent branch as pharmaceutical sciences, mainly through the acquisition of the wealth of knowledge, research and a vast array of drugs and therapeutic remedies. Unlike the other curricula, pharmacy is a product as well as service related discipline, increasing its scope many-fold.

Pharmacy is involved in all the stages related to a drug, from its discovery, development, action, safety, formulation, use, quality control, packaging, storage, marketing, etc. Thus, today's pharmacy professional is a "drug expert" in the real sense. The profession of pharmacy has transformed into a hub for the "Global Health care" and evolved as a multidisciplinary, versatile prospectus.

The drugs and pharma industry is a multibillion-dollar business. In the rapidly changing global scenario and the implementation of GATT and TRIPS in India, now a matter of only a couple of years, the pharmaceutical industry and professionals will play a vital role in shaping up our national economy. This new decade is thus, bound to have an ever-growing demand of pharmacy professionals not only in the country, but even worldwide. Anticipating this demand the government has taken special steps to boost this unique discipline having a blend of both technology, as well as, health sciences.

Some of the Indian universities like NIPER, Chandigarh, BITS-Pilani, University of Pune, Vadodara, etc. have given a special status to the pharmacy education by setting up a separate faculty of pharmaceutical sciences. In India, Pharmacy Education is a two-tier system. After 12th Science of State Board one can opt for any of the two courses, namely Diploma (D Pharm) and Degree (B Pharm). However, the Diploma Students can also be included in Degree course directly in Second Year B Pharm. However, in the coming years the Government and Pharmacy Council of India is planning to abolish the D Pharm course and make B Pharm, the minimum qualification for any individual to become a registered pharmacist.

The regulatory bodies for pharmacy colleges are, namely All India Council of Technical Education (AICTE), Pharmacy Council of India (PCI) and the respective university to which the college is affiliated to. Today pharmacy education like the pharmaceutical industry is also in the process of globalization. In order to have uniformity in course contents, requisite standards of education, technical faculty, facilities and infrastructure at international levels, colleges are going for accreditation and certifications from internationally approved regulating agencies like NBA.

Career Opportunities

A career in pharmacy, open out a view full of opportunities leading to a golden future for a young career aspirant. The job opportunities, working conditions, job satisfaction and monetary benefits are excellent.

The various career, a pharmacy professional can opt, are discussed below.

Production and Manufacturing

A pharmacy professional can work as a production person (chemist, officer, executive, manager, vice-president), involved in the production of bulk drug and intermediates or formulations and dosage forms. Industries in the cosmetics, soaps, toiletries segment also hire pharmacy professionals. Other segments where opportunities exist are the field of dental products. Production of biological and biotechnological products, surgical dressings, medical devices and equipment, ayurvedic/homoeopathic/unani medicines also involve the presence of pharmacy professionals in its production. Other areas where pharmacy professionals are required in production of veterinary medicine, perfumery, fragrances, and nutra-ceuticals.

Research and Development

This forms the heart of any industry, as it is the key to growth and nutrition. Mainly M Pharm and PhDs are in a great demand in the various areas of pharmaceutical R&D. Other areas where professionals are required, are:

- **New drug discovery research (NDDR):** Discovering a new drug has assumed prime importance in the post-GATT era.

- **Process and development (P&D):** One of the important areas in bulk drugs industry is developing workable processes for the manufacture of drugs and intermediates for their commercial production.

- **Formulation and development (F&D):** The success of any pharma company lies in the quality of its products, i.e. its formulations and dosage forms.

- **Clinical trials, bioequivalence studies, toxicological studies:** These are some of the areas of clinical research which are in high demand as they are involved in the systematic evaluation of potential drug substances prior to getting them approved by the authorities.

Analysis and Testing

Any drug or dosage form for human use has to be of excellent quality and purity, free from any impurities. The permitted limits of impurities, which either occurs through the manufacturing process, equipment, raw materials, handling or storage, are very strict. Therefore, quality control (QC) and quality assurance (QA) are the most integral areas of the drug and pharmaceutical industry. Highly specialized and trained staff is required to handle sensitive analytical procedures and sophisticated equipment. MPharm and PhDs in Pharm Analysis/Quality Assurance are highly preferred for this job.

Marketing

Any business is incomplete without the marketing and sales aspect, as the universal fact is that anything produced has to be sold. The Pharma: Sales and Marketing is a highly technical field and offers excellent opportunities for the pharmacy graduates. Additional qualification like MBA adds to their arsenal. An aspirant of a highly bright future can enter through various openings like starting his own retail or wholesale drug store or becoming a professional sales representative (known as medical Sales Representative or MR) to the levels of

International Marketing and Exports. The financial rewards and perks are the best.

Hospital Pharmacy

Another opening for a Pharmacy professional is as a "Registered Pharmacist" in the hospitals or drug stores. This is a very sought after professional especially in countries like the USA and Canada. The trend is already set in many hospitals in the country. This is a key position and the pharmacist plays an important role from preparing prescription to the patient's medial history after the Medical doctor has diagnosed the disease. The pharmacist is the best-informed qualified drug expert whose advice is sought by everybody regarding the dosage, incompatibilities and side effects of drugs.

Community Pharmacy

This concept, which is already very old in developed Western countries, is rapidly catching up the health care service in our country. Through the services of community pharmacy a pharmacist becomes a vital link between the patients and the products, i.e. drugs. The pharmacist also serves a vital link between the patients and other health care professionals, especially the medical experts.

- Counseling the patients regarding the use of the drugs and dosage forms
- Providing up-to-date information on drugs/dosage forms to the patients, as well as, medical staff.
- Maintaining patient records and history.
- Involved in the usage of self-diagnostic kits by the patients for disorders like diabetes, hypertension, etc.
- Providing supply of home care dosage forms.

Academics

Excellent opportunities for the professionals are available in teaching profession also. As per the AICTE norms the minimum entry-level qualification as lecturer is M Pharm. This is a profession associated with job satisfaction and social status as teaching is considered to be noble profession. The higher posts in the hierarchy and Senior Lecturer, Reader, Assistant Professor, Professor, Principal, etc. The emoluments are satisfactory.

Besides teaching academic related opportunities involve positions on research posts and training programs.

Regulatory Affairs

Locally the foods and drugs control administration (FDA) is the main regulatory body governing and implementing the rules and regulations for the Drug and Pharma industry. The FDA has state branches and sub-branches all over the country. The job opportunities for pharmacy graduates are excellent and range from the levels of a Drug Inspector (DI), Senior DI, Deputy Drug Controller, Assistant Drug Controller, Drug Controller and finally DCI (Drug Controller of India). This is highly respected and sought after profession. A graduate in pharmacy is the minimum eligibility.

With globalization process reaching out to India, the geographical barriers have become outdated. Any country will have to compete and trade globally in order to progress and survive in the years to come. The major drugs and pharma Companies have realized this fact and have stepped into the global area of competitive trade. If an Indian manufacturer wants to sell his drug or formulation to a foreign country it is mandatory that he has to fulfill all the statutory requirements laid by the regulatory authorities of that country. Also, his product needs to be perfectly as per the specifications laid down by the concerned regulatory authority. Thus, in order to enter into trade with the foreign countries it is compulsory to get the necessary approvals and sanctions as per the formats given by local regulatory authorities, e.g. approvals to be obtained from USFDA for the USA, TGA for Australia and New Zealand, MCA and MCM for the UK and the European countries and ICH guidelines going to be uniform for international levels.

Since, the business involved is worth multibillion dollars; this branch has assumed tremendous significance and is bound to grow enormously, in the Post-GATT era. Many big players in the drugs and pharmaceutical field has already established separate Regulatory Affairs Departments in a their companies. Regulatory experts are thus in a great demand.

Similarly, patents and trademarks, IPR. Experts are also in high demand as far as the pharmaceutical industry is concerned.

Documentation, Library Information Services and Pharmaceutical Journalism

The regulatory affairs as well as, patenting processes and issues involve a lot of documentation work to be done and submitted to the concerned regulatory authorities, in a highly specialized and technical manner. Pharmacy professionals are again fitting in the bill. Most of the major Indian pharmaceutical companies have established separate documentation departments with a highly technical and skilled staff for this purpose.

Similarly, the R&D and QC Departments of the Pharmaceutical Companies need a wealth of technical information, which needs to be updated regularly, in order to match the pace of global competition. Therefore, library information services are another field in much demand as far as the pharmaceutical industry is concerned. Furthermore, with the advent and boom of the Information Technology, Bioinformatics and Electronic Data Retrieval Systems, this field is already scaling new heights.

Pharma: Journalism is another area filled with a great potentialities. This requires specialist technical personnel like pharmacy graduates on the editorial staff to cover the various aspects. There is already a very profitable business in this field.

Consultancy

This is an ideal opportunity for highly technical and experienced pharmacy professionals to earn handsomely as self-employed entrepreneurs, even after the age of retirement. Consultancy services in pharmacy are offered in various fields against very attractive financial fees

- Regulatory affairs
- Documentation
- Approvals
- Manufacturing processes
- Analytical series

- Research
- Market surveys and sales promotion
- Information retrieval
- Data management

Opportunities Abroad

Golden opportunities galore for qualified pharmacy professionals in various courtiers including the USA, Canada, European Countries like UK, France, Germany, African Countries like S. Africa, Nigeria, Yemen, Gulf Countries like Saudi Arabia, Kuwait, South East Asian Countries like Singapore, Korea, Japan, etc. and the Australian Continent including N. Zealand.

There are plenty of higher education and research opportunities in the developed Western countries along with excellent job openings. The pharmaceutical career is one of the highest rewarding careers in these countries.

The monetary job benefits abroad are highly exciting, job profiles in African Countries like Nigeria, Yemen and Gulf Countries like Saudi Arabia, Kuwait mainly as pharmacists in drug stores and hospitals.

In developed Western countries the job opportunities are manifold and almost in any one of the ten vocations discussed above.

INTRODUCTION TO PHARMACOPOEIA

The term Pharmacopoeia comes from Greek word *"Pharmakon"* meaning 'drug' and *"Poein"* meaning 'make', and the combination means any recipe or formula or other standard required to make or prepare a drug.

"*Pharmacopoeia (literally, the art of the drug compounder), in its modern technical sense, is a book containing directions for the identification of samples and the preparation of compound medicines, and published by the authority of a government or a medical or pharmaceutical society. The name has also been applied to similar compendiums issued by private individuals*".

History of Pharmacopoeia

Some of the earliest pharmacopoeia books were written by Muslim physicians. These included *The Canon of Medicine* of

Avicenna in the 1020s and other pharmacopoeia books by Abu-Rayhan Biruni in the 11th century, Ibn Zuhr (Avenzoar) in the 12th century (and printed in 1491), and Ibn Baytar in the 14th century. The first work of the kind published under government authority appears to have been that of Nuremberg in 1542; a passing student named Valerius Cordus showed a collection of medical receipts, which he had selected from the writings of the most eminent medical authorities, to the physicians of the town. An earlier work, known as the *Antidotarium Florentinum*, had been published under the authority of the college of medicine of Florence. The term *pharmacopoeia* was first given by **Dr A. Foes** in 1561 in a work published at Basel.

The term 'Pharmacopoeia' was first used in 1580 in a book on drug standards printed in Bergamo, Italy. After that a number of national pharmacopoeia were published by various European Pharmacopoeias the London, the Edinburgh and the Dublin. Until 1617 such drugs and medicines as were in common use were sold in England by the apothecaries and grocers. The apothecaries obtained a separate charter and it was enacted that no grocer should keep an apothecary's shop. The preparation of physicians' prescriptions was thus confined to the apothecaries, this was than there responsibility to make and dispense medicines accurately, by the issue of a pharmacopoeia in May 1618 by the College of Physicians, and by the power which the wardens of the apothecaries received in common with the censors of the College of Physicians of examining the shops of apothecaries within 7 m of the London and destroying all the compounds which they found unfaithfully prepared. Then, the first authorized London Pharmacopoeia, was selected chiefly from the works of Mezue and Nicolaus de Salerno, but it was so full of errors that the whole edition was cancelled, and a fresh edition was published in the following December. At this period the compounds employed in medicine were often heterogeneous mixtures, some of which contained from 20 to 70, or more, ingredients, while a large number of samples were used in consequence of the same substance being supposed to possess different qualities according to the source from which it was derived. Although other editions of the London Pharmacopoeia were issued in 1621, 1632, 1639 and 1677, it was not until the edition of 1721, published under the guidance of Sir Hans Sloane, when all important alterations were made. In the edition published in 1788, the tendency to simplify was carried out to a much greater extent, and the extremely compound medicines which had formed the principal remedies of physicians for 2000 years were discarded, while a few powerful drugs which had been considered too dangerous to be included in the pharmacopoeia of 1765 were restored to their previous position. In 1809, the French chemical nomenclature was adopted, and in 1815, a corrected impression of the same was issued. Subsequent editions were published in 1824, 1836 and 1851.

Pharmacopoeia were official throughout the United Kingdom. Each pharmacopoeia described different strength and method of preparation for same preparation. Hence, there was a lot of confusion. To overcome this difficulty, the first British Pharmacopoeia came into existence in 1864. In the United States, the first pharmacopoeia was published in December 1820 both in English and in Latin. Later on a national formulary was also published in addition to USP (United States Pharmacopoeia). The object of first USP was to select from substances the ones which possess medicinal power, converted them into preparations of suitable composition in order to enhance their power to the maximum advantage. The first international pharmacopoeia was published by the World Health Organization in 1951 (volume 1) and in 1955 (volume 2).

These books are revised from time to time so as to introduce the latest information available as early as possible after they become established in order to introduce new products and to keep the size of book within reasonable limits it becomes necessary to omit certain less frequently used drugs and pharmaceutical adjuvant from each new edition of the book. Therefore in each new edition of these books certain new monographs are added while the older once are deleted.

For the preparation of these books the expert opinion of medical practitioners, teachers and pharmaceutical manu-facturers is obtained.

The drug compendia are classified as

1. Official compendia
2. Non-official compendia.

1. Official Compendia

Official compendia are the compilations of drugs and others related substances which are recognized as legal standards of purity, quality and strength by a government agency of respective countries of there origin.

Official compendia's include British Pharmacopoeia, British Pharmaceutical Codex, Indian Pharmacopoeia, the United States Pharmacopoeia, national formulary, the state pharmacopoeia of USSR and pharmacopoeia of other countries.

2. Non-official Compendia

The books other than official drug compendia which are used as secondary reference source for drugs and other related substances are known as non-official drug compendia. Example like Merck index, Remington's pharmaceutical sciences, etc.

The History of Pharmacopoeia of India

The Government of India through its letter No. 2338H(C)/43 dated 26 January, 1944 , directed the Drugs Technical Advisory Board to list the drugs in use in India, which are not mentioned in British Pharmacopoeia and also recommend the standards to be prescribed to maintain uniformity and the chemical tests to be used to establish identity and purity. The Government of India published the Indian Pharmacopoeial List in 1946, as a supplement to the British Pharmacopoeia. The term "list" in the title was "misleading" in that, the book not only contained a list of drugs which were of substantial medicinal value but also laid down standards. The Indian Pharmacopoeial list contained about 180 monographs and a no. of appendices prepared on the lines of the British Pharmacopoeia.

Approximately 100 monographs were on vegetable drug growing in India and on their galenicals. For example berberis, cannabis, ispaghula, rauwalfia, vasaka, digitalis, etc. were included in it. Similarly, several oils such as chaulmoogra, neem, and pudina, were included in it. The Pharmaceuticals and Drug Research Committee of the Council of Scientists and Industrial Research decided in February 1947 to compile a "Brochure" to highlight the information and clinical uses of the important indigenous drugs of India, in the form of a "codex". The first Indian pharmaceutical codex was published in 1953. The codex consist of two parts: The first part carried about 190 general monographs on natural products and drugs of vegetable and animal origin, and a few chemicals. The second part consisted of formulary of galenicals and other preparations.

After the publication of Indian Pharmacopoeial List, the government of India constituted an eleven-member Indian Pharmacopoeial Committee in 1948, in their notification No. F.1–1/48-DS dated 23rd November, 1948, for preparing the Pharmacopoeia of India. The tenure of the office of the members of committee was five year. It was extended by one year vide Government notification No. F.6–10/53-DS dated the 21st November, 1953. In compiling the monographs of the first Pharmacopoeia of India, help was taken from all available established scientific data in modern pharmacopoeia, such as British Pharmacopoeia, the United States Pharmacopoeia, International Pharmacopoeia, and from scientific institutions interested in drugs and pharmaceutical products. The first edition of Pharmacopoeia of India was compiled and then published in 1955.

Main Features of First Edition of Pharmacopoeia of India (1955)

1. The title of monograph was given in Latin language and abbreviated titles for use of prescription were given immediately below the Latin line.
2. The English title were also given below the abbreviation title.
3. The weights and measures were given in metric system.
4. All statements given in the individual monographs were considered as constitute standards for official substances.
5. Doses were expressed both in the metric system as well as in the English system.
6. A list of preparation was given at the end of some of the monographs.
7. The temperature was expressed in celsius.
8. The descriptive terms (very soluble, freely soluble, sparingly soluble, slightly soluble, very slightly soluble, practically insoluble) have been used where the exact solubility of a pharmacopoeial substance is not known.

The tenure of the Indian Pharmacopoeial Committee expired in 1954, and the Committee was reconstituted under the chairmanship of Dr BN Ghosh, Professor of Pharmacology, RG Kar Medical College, Calcutta. The Committee compiled a supplement to the first edition of the Indian Pharmacopoeia. The supplement was published in 1960. The composition of the committee was as follows:

1. Chairman 1
2. Members 11
3. Member Secretary 1
4. Assistant Secretary 1

A subcommitte was appointed by the committee to help in the compilation work, the following subcommittee were made.

1. Pharmacology and Bioassay Subcommittee.
2. Biological Product Subcommittee.
3. Antibodies, Vitamins and Hormones Subcommittee.
4. Pharmacognosy Subcommittee.
5. Pharmacy Subcommittee.
6. Pharmaceutical Subcommittee.
7. General Chemistry Subcommittee.
8. Analytical Subcommittee.
9. Physical Standards, Weights, Measures and Nomenclature Subcommittee.
10. Indian Medical Plants Subcommittee.

A coordination subcommittee consisting of the chairman and secretary of the Indian Pharmacopoeia Committee and the chairman of the various subcommittees was also constituted to coordinate the work of various subcommittees. The second edition of the pharmacopoeia of India was published in 1966 and later on its supplement was published in 1975.

Main Features of the Second Edition of Pharmacopoeia of India (1975)

1. The titles of monographs were changed from Latin to English.
2. The name of the drug was given first, e.g. injection of ranitidine has been changed to ranitidine injection.
3. Doses were expressed in the metric system only.

4. Solubility is expressed in parts of solvent per unit part of solute.
5. The preparations of a drug have been given immediately after the monographs on the parent drug.
6. For the detection of fungi apart from aerobic and anaerobic bacteria, the test for sterility was included.
7. New analytical techniques such as non-aqueous titrimetry, column chromatography, HPLC were added
8. In the monographs of "tablets" and "injection", a new subheading "usual strength" has been given to represent the strength of the tablet or injection.
9. Some drugs were renamed in this edition, e.g. 'acetylsalicylic acid 'has been changed to 'aspirin'.

The Government of India, Ministry of Health and Family Welfare, vide their resolution No. X 19014/1/77-D & MS, dated 30th June 1979, reconstituted the Indian Pharmacopoeia Committee for a period of five years for the preparation of the edition of Pharmacopoeia of India. The composition of the committee was as follows:

  i. Chairman 1
 ii. Members 13 from academic, research and industry.
iii. Member Secretary 1
iv. Assistant Secretary 1

The committee appointed the following subcommittees

1. Clinical Medicines and Pharmacology Subcommittee.
2. Biological Products and Bioassay Subcommittee.
3. Antibiotics Subcommittee.
4. Synthetic Drugs Subcommittee.
5. Medicinal Plants, Galenicals and Surgical-Dressing Subcommittee.
6. Chemicals and Sterile Products Subcommittee.
7. Parenteral and Sterile Products Subcommittee.
8. Non-parenteral Products Subcommittee.
9. Analytical Methods, Reagents, Diagnostic Aids and Containers Subcommittee.
10. Nomenclature and Formulae Subcommittee.

The Indian Pharmacopoeia Committee also constituted a "Working Group" for the purpose of preparing draft monographs and appendices, to examine the comments received on these from various sources and then make suitable recommendations to the committee.

The monographs, appendices and general notices are prepared by the "working Group" and finalized by the committee were then published in the form of third edition of Pharmacopoeia of India in 1985 by the Government of India.

Main Features of Third Edition of Pharmacopoeia of India (1985)

1. The newer analytical techniques like Flame Photometry, Flurimetry, Electrophoresis were introduced for certain analytical methods.
2. For certain tablets, dissolution test was introduced.
3. Disintegration test was modified regarding the design of the apparatus and method of testing.
4. Microbial limit test was prescribed for various pharmaceutical aids and oral liquid dosage form.
5. In spite of shivering response for rabbit the pyrogen test was introduced.
6. Gas liquid chromatography (GLC) was introduced for analytical purposes of alcohol concentration detection.
7. Ostwald viscometer was used to determine the viscosity.
8. The new appendix on "Water for Pharmaceutical Use" has been introduced for purified water, water for injection and sterile water for injection.
9. Drugs were renamed, e.g. 'acetylsalicylic acid' has been changed to 'aspirin'.
10. New drugs were added and some drugs were omitted from the third edition.

The Government of India, Ministry of Health and Family Welfare vide their resolution No. X19020/1/89-DMS and PFA dated 12th August 1991, reconstituted the Indian Pharmacopoeia Committee for a period of five years for the preparation of the fourth edition of pharmacopoeia of India. The composition of the committee was as follows:

1. Chairman 1
2. Members 18 in number representing academic, research and industry.

3. Member Secretary 1
4. Assistant Secretary 1

The committee appointed the subcommittees and working groups in order to expedite the preparation of the new edition of the Indian Pharmacopoeia.

The Monographs, Appendices and General Notes as prepared by the "Working Group" and finalized by the committee were then published in the form of fourth edition of the Pharmacopoeia of India in 1996 by the Government of India

Main Features of the Fourth Edition of Pharmacopoeia of India (1996)

1. It contains 1149 monographs and 123 appendices in two volumes.
2. It contains computer-generated structural formulae
3. Some titles were changed to include the more commonly accepted names, e.g. hyoscine hydrobromide for scopolamine hydrobromide.
4. Infrared and ultra-red adsorption spectrophotometric tests for identification of drug substance were added. The infrared reference spectra of a number of drug substances were also included in an appendix.
5. The high performance liquid chromatography (HPLC) has been widely used as a method to analyze many formulations which can otherwise be analyzed only by more difficult and less accurate method, e.g. biological assay of insulin has been replaced by HPLC.
6. Bacterial endotoxins test for pyrogens has been introduced.
7. A number of general monographs, e.g. eye drops; eye ointments, nasal preparation, oral liquids, pessaries, suppositories, etc. have been included.
8. A quantitative method for determining particulate matter in injectable preparations has been replaced by the qualitative test.
9. The specific biological assays and tests provided for vaccines; hormones, blood products and enzymes have been transferred to the individual monograph.
10. In the monograph of oral rehydration salts (ORS), ORS—bicarbonate formula was omitted due to its stability

problem, whereas ORS—citrate formula recommended by WHO is added.

British Pharmacopoeia

The British Pharmacopoeia (BP) is a collection of quality standards for the UK medicinal substances. It is used by individuals and organizations involved in pharmaceutical research, development, manufacturing and testing. The British Pharmacopoeia is an important statutory component in the control of medicines which complements and assists the licensing and inspection processes of the Medicines and Health care products Regulatory Agency (MHRA) of the United Kingdom. It is published every year.

The British Pharmacopoeia is published by the Health Ministers of the United Kingdom on the recommendation of the Commission on Human Medicines in accordance with Section 99(6) of the Medicines Act, 1968 and notified in draft to the European Commission in accordance with Directive 98/34/EEC.

In 1907, the British Pharmacopoeia was supplemented by the British Pharmaceutical Codex, which gave information on drugs and other pharmaceutical substances not included in the BP, and provided standards for these.

The first publication of British Pharmacopoeia was in 1864 and has grown throughout the world. It is now used in over 100 countries. Australia and Canada are two of the countries that have adopted the BP as their national standard alongside the UK, and in other countries (e.g. Korea) it is recognized as an internationally acceptable standard. The BP is prepared by the Pharmacopoeial Secretariat working in collaboration with the BP Laboratory, the British Pharmacopoeia Commission (BPC) and its Expert Advisory Groups (EAG) and Advisory Panels. The development of pharmacopoeial standards receives input from relevant industries, hospitals, academia, professional bodies and governmental sources, both within and outside the UK. The BP Laboratory provides analytical and technical support to the British Pharmacopoeia.

The current edition of the British Pharmacopoeia comprises six volumes, which contain nearly 3,000 monographs for drug substances, excipients and formulated preparation, together with supporting General Notices, Appendices (test methods, reagents, etc.) and Reference Spectra used in the practice of medicine, all comprehensively indexed and cross-referenced for easy reference.

BP volumes I and II contain

- Medicinal substances

BP volume III contains

- Formulated preparations
- Blood related preparations,
- Immunological products,
- Radiopharmaceutical preparations
- Surgical materials
- Homeopathic preparations

BP volume IV contains

- Appendices
- Infrared reference spectra
- Index

BP volume V contains

- British Pharmacopoeia (veterinary)

BP volume VI (CD-ROM version) contains

- British Pharmacopoeia
- British Pharmacopoeia (veterinary)
- British approved names

The BP is available as a printed volume and electronically in both online and CD-ROM versions, the electronic products use sophisticated search techniques to locate information quickly. For example, pharmacists referring to a monograph can immediately link to other related substances and appendices referenced in the content by using 1,30,000+ hypertext links within the text.

The major functions of BP are

1. Development of new pharmacopoeial monographs
2. Development and validation of qualitative and quantitative test methods for new BP monograph specifications

3. Refining and revalidating test methods for existing BP monographs.

British Pharmaceutical Codex

It was in 1903 that the council of the pharmaceutical society of Great Britain decided to prepare a reference book for the use of medical practitioners and dispensing pharmacists. The first edition of the British Pharmaceutical Codex was published in 1907. The subsequent revisions of this codex were published in 1911, 1923, 1934, 1949, 1954, 1959, 1963, 1968, and 1973.

On the request of British Pharmacopoeia Commission, the council of the pharmaceutical society agreed in 1959 for the publication of codex to coincide with that of the British Pharmacopoeia, so that these two books, i.e. British Pharmaceutical Codex and British Pharmacopoeia should come into effect on the same dates.

The British Pharmaceutical Codex differs from British Pharmacopoeia in that:

1. It contains many new drugs and preparations; some were included in advance, which were in the pipeline of clinical trials or synthesis.
2. It provides standards for drugs, surgical dressings and pharmaceutical preparations not included in the British Pharmacopoeia.
3. It provides information on the actions and uses of drugs, their undesirable effects, precautions and the treatment of poisoning.
4. It contains formulae, method of preparation, dose, container and storage conditions of majority of pharmaceutical preparations, e.g. mixtures, powders, eye drops, ear drops, liniments, lotions, ointments, creams, pastes, suppositories, etc.

United States Pharmacopoeia

The United States Pharmacopoeia is an official public standards—setting authority for all prescription and over-the-counter medicines and other health care products manufactured or sold in the United States. USP also sets recognized standards for food ingredients and dietary supplements. These standards help to ensure the quality, purity, strength, and consistency of products made for public consumption. USP's standards are recognized and used in more than 130 countries around the globe. The United States Pharmacopoeia and the National Formulary (USP-NF) are recognized as official compendia and are used as reference books for determining the strength, quality, purity, packaging and labeling of drugs and other related articles.

The United States Pharmacopoeia was originally published in 1820 under the authority of the United States Pharmacopoeial convention and the National Formulary was published in 1888 under the guidance of the American Pharmaceutical Association. In 1974, the National Formulary was purchased by the United States Pharmacopoeial convention and from 1980 onwards only one official book of drug standards was published under the heading, the United States Pharmacopoeia and the National formulary (USP-NF).

USP is a non-governmental, not-for-profit public health organization whose independent, volunteer experts work under strict conflict-of-interest rules to set its scientific standards. USP's work is aided by the participation and oversight of volunteers representing pharmacy, medicine, and other health care professions as well as academia, government, the pharmaceutical and food industries, health plans, and consumer organizations.

Main Features of USP

1. Product quality—standards and verification

USP establishes documentary and reference standards to ensure quality medicines, food ingredients, and other health care products. Prescription and over-the-counter medicines available in the United States must, by federal law, meet USP's public standards, where such standards exist. Many other countries require the use of high-quality standards such as USP's to assure the quality of medicines and related products. USP also conducts verification programs for dietary supplement ingredients. Much like food ingredients, USP's standards for dietary supplements have no legal recognition in the United States, but involve independent testing and review to verify ingredient and product integrity, purity, and potency for manufacturers who choose to participate.

2. Health care information

USP develops information relating to various aspects of drug use and disseminates this information to practitioners, pharmacists, and others who make decisions about health care around the world. Significant among USP's health care information initiatives is the development of a drug classification system that Medicare Prescription Drug Benefit Plans may use to develop their formularies. USP also partners with the US. Agency for International Development, the World Health Organization and others in worldwide projects that help to assure drug quality and proper drug use in many developing countries.

3. Patient safety

USP operates two programs to promote safer care of patients who take medications and stay in hospitals. The Medication Errors Reporting Program allows health care professionals to directly report medication errors to USP. MEDMARX®, an internet-based medication error and adverse drug reaction reporting program, is designed for use in hospitals and health systems. USP also uses its knowledge base to provide information that supports the health care community in the research and development of patient safety initiatives.

4. Drug quality and information

USP's Drug Quality and Information (USP DQI) Program is a cooperative agreement with the United States Agency for International Development (USAID). The USP DQI program has established a presence in USAID-priority countries on four continents advancing strategies to improve drug quality and the appropriate use of drugs.

The four main programs that USP promotes

1. Ensuring drug quality by working with local governments, USAID missions, the World Health Organization (WHO), and other partners to evaluate a country's readiness and capacity to provide necessary drug quality assurance.

2. Providing continuing education for physicians, pharmacists and nurses in drug information and pharmacovigilance to help improve drug dispensing and ensure competence and accountability.

3. Developing and disseminating evidence-based drug and therapeutic information through targeted drug and therapeutic information materials for health care providers based on specific needs.

4. Establishing regional and international cooperation through USP's system of open conferences, internet-based communications, and regular publications.

USP's Global Presence

Activities at USP are focused on promoting the public health by disseminating authoritative standards and information for over-the-counter medicines, dietary supplements, food ingredients and other health care technologies, and related practices used to maintain and improve health and promote optimal health care delivery around the world.

The International Pharmacopoeia

The International Pharmacopoeia (Ph. Int.), is issued by the World Health Organization.

The aim is to achieve a wide global uniformity of quality specifications for selected pharmaceutical products, excipients, and dosage forms.

High priority is given to medicines that are important to WHO health programs, and which may not appear in any other pharmacopoeias, e.g. new antimalarial drugs.

The International Pharmacopoeia (Ph. Int.) comprises a collection of quality specifications for pharmaceutical substances (active ingredients and excipients) and dosage forms together with supporting general methods of analysis that is intended to serve as source material for reference or adaptation by any WHO Member State wishing to establish pharmaceutical requirements.

The activities related to the International Pharmacopoeia are an essential element in the overall quality control and assurance of pharmaceuticals contributing to the safety and efficacy of medicines. The International Pharmacopoeia recognizes the needs of specific disease programmes and the essential medicines nominated under these programmes; it is based primarily on those substances included in the current WHO Model List of Essential Medicines. The work on the International Pharmacopoeia is carried out in collaboration with members of the WHO Expert Advisory Panel on the International Pharmacopoeia and Pharmaceutical Preparations and with other specialists. The process involves consultation of and input from WHO Member States and drug regulatory authorities.

PRACTICE QUESTIONS
Very Short Answer Type Questions

1. What does the term "Pharmacon" means?
2. Name the scientist who made major contribution in the development of pharmacy profession.
3. Define the term Pharmacopoeia.
4. In which year was the first British Pharmacopoeia published?
5. Give the year of publication of first USP.
6. In which year did the first pharmacopoeia of India come out?
7. How many monographs are there in Indian Pharmacopoeial List?
8. When was the first International Pharmacopoeial List published?
9. Who was publisher of Indian Pharmacopoeia?
10. When was Indian Pharmacopoeial List published?
11. In which year the various editions of the pharmacopoeia of India come out?
12. When was the first Indian Phrarmaceutical Codex published?
13. When was the term "Pharmacopoeia" used for the first time?
14. When was the First International Pharmacopoeia published?

SHORT ANSWER TYPE QUESTIONS

1. Define the term Pharmacopoeia.
2. Name the various pharmacopoeias commonly used in India.
3. Name the various standards reference books on pharmacy in common use in our country.
4. Give the reasons for the publication of International Pharmacopoeia by WHO.
5. Why did publication of Indian pharmacopoeial List in 1946 became necessary?
6. Differentiate between official and non-official compendia.

LONG ANSWER TYPE QUESTIONS

1. Describe in detail the various stages, which ultimately led to the development of first pharmacopoeia of India.
2. Write in brief about history of pharmacopoeia.
3. Discuss briefly the scope of pharmacy.
4. Write in detail about the origin and development of pharmacy.
5. Give the salient features of the second edition of pharmacopoeia of India.
6. What are the salient features of the third edition of pharmacopoeia of India?
7. Why did the publication of British Pharmacopoeia became necessary?
8. Give, in brief, the history of the pharmacopoeia of India.
9. Differentiate between BP and BPC.
10. Write in brief about the International Pharmacopoeia of India.
11. Write in brief about the United States Pharmacopoeia of India.

OBJECTIVE TYPE QUESTIONS
Multiple Type Questions

1. The new edition of British Pharmacopoeia is published after every:
   (1) 4 years   (2) 5 years
   (3) 6 years   (4) Alt. year

2. The first edition of the Pharmacopoeia of India was published in:
   (1) 1947   (2) 1955
   (3) 1966   (4) 1946

3. The supplement to second edition of pharmacopoeia of India was published in:
   (1) 1981   (2) 1975
   (3) 1985   (4) 1966

4. The first USP was published in:
   (1) 1820   (2) 1830
   (3) 1845   (4) 1855

5. The Indian Pharmacopoeial List was published as a supplement to:
   (1) British Pharmacopoeia   (2) USP
   (3) Pharmacopoeia of India   (4) IPC

6. *"De Materia Medica"* was written by ....

7. ....……….. is the father of medicine.

8. ………….. made major contribution for *"Galenic Pharmacy"*

9. Father of ayurveda is ……….....................................…..

10. FDA stands for ……………....................................………

11. AICTE stands for ……………...................................…...

12. PCI stands for ……………...................................…......

13. TRIPS stands for ……………...............................……...

14. DI stands for ……………….................................………

15. ICH stands for ……………...................................……...

16. Term pharmacopoeia comes from .... word .... meaning .... and poein meaning ....

17. The term pharmacopoeia was first given by .... in his work published at ....

18. Match the following:

Name of the scientist	Time period
1. Hippocrates	a. First century AD
2. Dioscorides	b. a.c 130–200 AD
3. Galen	c. 1793–1541 AD
4. Paracelsus	d. a.c 460–377 BC

ANSWERS

1. (4)
2. (2)
3. (3)
4. (1)
5. (1)
6. Dioscorides
7. Hippocrates
8. Claudius Galen
9. Charak
10. Food and Drug Administration Act
11. All India Council for Technical Education
12. Pharmacy Council of India
13. Trade related intellectual property and rights
14. Drug inspector
15. International conference on hormonisation
16. Greek, pharmacon, drug, to make
17. Dr. A. Foes, Basel
18. 1-d, 2-a, 3-b, 4-c

2

Pharmaceutical Additives

The human body is endowed with five antenna dishes which receive different signals from the environments and feed them to the brain for processing and commands. Three of these are actuated by energy and two by chemical molecules. The senses of sight, hearing and touch arise due to light waves, sonic waves and pressure respectively. The taste and odor are stimulated by chemical molecules.

History records that medicaments have been notorious for bad sensual characteristics throughout although consciousness, to make them more palatable and acceptable to the senses prevailed. If the medicine was bitter and had to be taken there was no alternative to it. But in modern age the acceptability of dosage from by the senses or its organoleptic properties are considered very important qualities of the product and formulator cannot afford to lose sight of this fact. Amongst the important organoleptic characteristics which are manipulated to make dosage form more pleasant are:

1. Color
2. Taste and
3. Odor.

COLORING AGENT

Physically speaking color consists of the sensation produced when visible rays between the wavelength of 400 and 800 nm strike the retina. When the admixture of all visible wavelengths constituting *'white light'* falls on an object there could be following alternatives:

a. Practically all wavelengths are absorbed—then the substance will appear black

b. Practically all wavelengths are reflected back—then the substance will appear white

c. Neither any wavelength is absorbed or reflected back—then the substance will appear colorless

d. Some wavelengths are absorbed while others are reflected back—then the substance will appear colored.

The color of any given substance is determined by wavelengths that it reflects. A substance appears red when it is bathed in white light and reflects the red wavelengths absorbing other wavelengths. In ancient times, the chief sources of color were the three natural kingdoms, namely mineral, plant and animal kingdom.

The mineral colors were composed of material such as ferric oxide (red and yellow), lead chromate, prussian blue, vermillion, titanium dioxide, carbon black, etc. These colors were used for painting, coloring of chinaware and coloration of lotions. But these days hardly any color of mineral origin is used for such purposes.

Plants were the most important sources of colors in ancient times. Notable colors of plant world were alizarin, anthocyanins, carotenoids, chlorophyll, flavones, etc. Indigo was a fascinating rage and during British times India also had several indigo producing units. Alizarin obtained from *Rubia tinctorum* is still used in one form or other. Beta carotene extracted from carrots is yellow and has been used for coloring margarine. Flavones like the riboflavin, hesperidin, rutin, etc. are all yellow and when present in formulation impart their color. Saffron which is highly priced and along with color possess a very delicate and acceptable flavor is used, especially in India, for coloring and flavoring food delicacies. Cudbear and red saunders are also derived from plants.

The animal world has been comparatively a minor source of colors. *Tyrian blue* was obtained by oxidizing a colorless secretion from glands of snails. Cochineal, an insect containing a bright red color, carminic acid, figured in the formula of Tr. card co. some while ago.

Synthetic colors were discovered with accidental breaking of thermometer by Perkin in 1856 while attempting to synthesize quinine. He obtained dyes by oxidation of aniline containing para and orthotoluidines as impurities. Perkin's discovery became a major breakthrough in world of colors. From that day onwards man learnt to create colors in test tubes and his dependence on nature for colors became nearly a closed chapter. The early synthetic colors were evolved from aniline and were popular as aniline colors. Since then the color chemistry has made a tremendous progress and now it is known various structures have chromophoric qualities. All synthetic colors are not fit for human consumption and hence a limited range which is non-toxic is specified for coloring foods, drugs, etc. The list of *'permitted'* colors is published under the authority of government. The following is the list of colors permitted under Drugs and Cosmetics Act, 1940.

1. *Natural colors:* Annato, carotene, chlorophyll, cochineal, curcumin, red and yellow oxides of iron, titanium dioxide.

2. *Artificial colors:* Caramel

3. *Coaltar colors:*

    • *Black*: Naphthol blue black 20470

    • *Blue*: Brilliant blue FCS 42090

    Indigocarmine 73015

    • *Brown*: Resorcin brown 20170

    • *Yellow*: Tartrazine 19140

    Sunset yellow FCF 15185

    Quinoline yellow SS 4700

    • *Green*: Fast green FCF 42053

    Quinazoline green 61565

    Green S 44090

    Alizarin cyanine green F 61570

    • *Orange*: Orange G 16230

    • *Red*: Amaranth IN 16185

    Erythrosin 45430

    Ponceaux 4R 16255

    Sudan III 26100

Carminosine 14720

Fast red E 16045

4. *Lakes*: These are those colors in which dyes are absorbed generally on aluminum hydroxide. The lakes consist of 15 to 40% of adsorbed dyes and are insoluble in water.

Desirable Characteristics of a Coloring Agent

1. It should be harmless to body and should have no toxic effect
2. It should be readily soluble in water.
3. Its color imparting capacity should be high, i.e. very small amount of color is required to give sufficient color.
4. It should be stable over a wide range of temperature, humidity and other atmospheric conditions.
5. It should not be affected by redox reactions as well as it should be stable over a wide range of pH.
6. It should be inert with respect to the other excipients, additives and active ingredient.
7. It should be readily available, inexpensive.
8. It should be free from objectionable taste and odour.
9. It should have a high shelf life, i.e. it can be stored for a longer duration of time.
10. It should give good psychological effect.

Choice of Colors for Formulations

Choice of color for a formulation may be a difficult decision for any formulator. First of all he has to decide on a shade and then fix up for the quantity to be incorporated. In deciding the kind of color the parameters cannot be clearly demarcated and sensitivity of judgment would be the best thing to rely upon. For instance, if an oral preparation is being formulated the colors that are associated with choice of food may be the most acceptable one. Red color with its shades of variations is very much accepted in foods. Yellow and green probably comes next. A blue or black may not be very much appealing. The pharmaceutical formulator can take cue from these hints in deciding upon color. Further, one has to keep in mind the harmonious blending of the color and the flavor.

If the flavor is that of lemon the color should also be lemon. If the flavor be rose, pink color will go with it best. Yet another consideration that often weights upon formulator is the personal preference of their costumer population.

For pharmaceutical products, especially solid dosage forms like tablets pastel shades are preferred because they show less of mottling than darker shades. The colors are also used in form of lakes which consist of dyes absorbed generally on aluminium hydroxide. The lakes consist of 15 to 40% of adsorbed dyes and are insoluble in water.

A new concept which is coming up is that of non-adsorbable polymeric colors which are also known as **ploydyes**. These colors are prepared by incorporation of biologically stable chromophores into non-degradable and non-absorbable polymeric chains. These colors are not absorbed in the GIT and as such do not constitute toxicity hazards. Polydyes are readily soluble and can be dry blended, spray dried emulsified, etc. These dyes are becoming popular as colorants for the foods as well. Lakes can be formed by adsorbing ploydyes on alumina up to 70 to 80%.

Incorporation of Colors

So far as the liquid products are concerned incorporation of colors present no problem since colors get dissolved in the vehicle and the product would be uniformly colored. However, incorporation of colors in solid dosage forms may be set with many problems. If the color to be incorporated in the dosage form like tablets are water soluble the best way may be to dissolve the same in water which is to be used for granulation as such or along with adhesives. This may ensure uniform distribution of color in the granulation but possibility of mottling during drying cannot be overlooked. Lake dyes give mottling on lesser occasions. Soluble dyes should first be adsorbed onto materials like calcium sulfate. 5 to 10% of MCC may prevent migration of dye during drying and consequent mottling.

Another established method is to adsorb dye onto materials like starch, lactose, etc. from aqueous or alcoholic solutions and use these colored materials in processing the tablets. Yet another possibility is to dry blend colors with one of the excipients prior to final admixture of the solid ingredients. Lake colors are dry blended in this fashion.

After having decided upon a shade for a particular preparation the next question arises its proportion. There are no hard and fast rules about the quantity of colors for different preparations but some guidelines are now available which form a very practical starting point. The general hints for quantities are liquids (solutions): 0.0001 to 0.001%, powders: 0.1%.

These guidelines are approximate indications and exact percentage has to be decided by trial and error. The dye in pharmaceutical preparations should be added in such amounts as would not produce permanent strains on any fabric.

The permitted colors are chiefly sodium salts and are as such anionic in nature. Some ions like Ca, Mg Al, etc. tend to form insoluble compounds with the permitted dyes. Changes in pH are also known to have resulted in change in color. Acids tend to release insoluble form of colors. Since concentrations of colors are generally low no precipitates are evident.

FLAVORING AGENTS

The flavor of a pharmaceutical formulation is a very important characteristic so much that then very success or failure of a commercial product can be interlinked with the quality of its flavor. In the traditional context the term flavor was equated with odorific qualities of a product though in the modern concept a flavor includes initial impact, mouth feel and after impact of the preparations.

The odorific qualities of a material depend up on its volatility in the warm and moist environment of mouth and its consequent interaction with olfactory cleft, a one centimeter square piece of tissue situated in the nasal chamber. Different substances give different perception and in the past the smell scientist have attempted at classification of odors. It has also been established that the sense of smell is a chemical sense and the odorific qualities of a compound depends upon its chemical structure.

Flavoring of a Pharmaceutical Products

Since flavors of pharmaceutical products are of a great significance in their marketing, the formula development man must adopt a rational approach in deciding flavor for a given product. Until recently the practice was to incorporate some natural flavor such as clove, eucalyptus, lemon, mint, orange, wintergreen, etc. in preparations meant for oral administration and flavors such as jasmine, lavender, rose, etc. for products meant for external use. These flavors did make the preparations acceptable but the entire approach is very different now.

These days the very first step is to evaluate the drug in its pure form with respect to its aroma, basic taste, mouth effects and overall impression. Simultaneously the intensity of these fundamental attributes is assessed. In case the drug has unacceptable taste an attempt is made to mask the same by techniques such as encapsulation, adsorption, spray congealing, ion-exchange, etc. However, if the taste of a drug is not very bad or alternately if it is to be incorporated in low dose this step may be done away with.

Thereafter the various additives should be decided upon keeping an eye on the ultimate flavor of the product. Sometimes it is possible to select adjuvants which not only mask the bad odor but which definitely give a good flavor. Then the drugs and adjuvants should be put together to produce samples of the unflavored product. At this stage it may be worthwhile using the services of an experienced flavor chemist. Nowadays many organizations specialize in flavors and as such pharmaceutical formulators need not exert themselves to select a flavor for their product. The flavor chemist can be supplied some samples of the unflavored formulations and requested to suggest suitable flavor for it. It will be useful to supply the basic data to the flavor chemist in the following format:

1. Name, structure, subjective taste, mouth feel, incompatibilities, stability data, etc. of the drug.
2. Broad therapeutic category of the drug whether it is antacid, multivalent formulation, antiseptic, cold remedy, etc.
3. The adjuvants proposed to be used.
4. Patient category whether children, adults or old people.
5. Preference of flavor.

The entire business of flavoring a product is so very intricate that only experts with long experiences can deliver right goods. The flavor should ultimately be in consonance with the taste as well as the color of the product (Tables 2.1 and 2.2). They should also cater to specific liking of patient population. Some guidelines in this respect are given below:

Table 2.1: Matches between tastes and flavors

Taste	Flavor/flavors
Alkaline	Mint, chocolate , vanilla, custard
Acid (sour)	Lemon, orange, anise, liquorice, raspberry, cherry, strawberry
Bitter	Anise, mint, fennel, chocolate, spicy, cherry
Metallic	Grape, lemon, burgundy
Salty	Citrus flavors, maple, raspberry, fruity, melon
Sweet	Fruity, vanilla, maple, honey

Table 2.2: Matching flavors and colors

Flavors	Colors
Raspberry, cherry, strawberry, apple, rose	Pink to red
Chocolate, honey, molasses, walnut, caramel	Brown
Lemon, lime, orange, custard, cherry	Yellow to orange
Banana, mint, pistachio	Green
Mint, vanilla, spearmint, jasmine, banana	White to off white
Grape, liquorice, violet	Violet or purple
Blueberry, mixed fruit, plum, liquorice	Blue

So far as patient population preferences are concerned there can be no universal rule of thumb approach since preferences may vary from one group to another. In general, however, children like very sweet flavors and so do people of geriatric group. Children prefer cherry, grape, orange, mint, etc., while older group may prefer flavors like orange, cherry, burgundy, etc. Adult preferences are vanilla, strawberry, mint, etc. Very string flavors as a rule should be avoided.

Marketed form of Flavors

At one time the flavors for pharmaceutical products consisted of volatile oils like anise, clove, fennel, lemon, orange, wintergreen, oils or of their separated fractions, such as thymol, menthol, camphor, etc. However, in recent times the flavors are also marketed as *spray dried powders* or adsorbed powders. The spray dried flavors are produced by emulsification of naturally occurring volatile oils using acacia, dextrin, etc. as the emulsifying agents followed by spray drying of the resultant emulsion. This technique produces very fine powders with low bulk density. However, it should be notice that spray drying may cause volatilization of the flavor oils to a small extent and may also modify the flavor note slightly. Generally the oil content of spray dried powders is around 20%.

In the adsorbed powders the flavoring material are adsorbed on materials like silica gel at room or very slightly elevated temperatures. The adsorbed powders may contain up to 70% of flavoring substance in contrast of 20% in case of spray dried powders. Generally the aroma of the adsorbed powders is no different from the original flavoring material because processing does not involve any drastic conditions like high temperatures. The latest marketed flavors are the microencapsulated beads. These products are catching up in spite of their high cost. The microencapsulated beads forms are generally prepared by coacervation. These are available as free flowing powders.

These newer forms of flavors are more suited for solid dosage forms for internal use because of ease of incorporation.

Storage of Flavors

The flavors in the modern forms may have to be stored for some time before being used. It is essential that during this period there is no qualitative change in them. The flavors obtained from a flavor company should be stored at a low temperature (15–30°C) and at a place where the relative humidity range is below 45%. In spite of all precautionary measures the flavors do not remain healthy beyond 12 months in the sense that there might be some change in their aroma or intended flavor quality. Normally flavors should be stocked in polythene bags enclosed in heavy plastic bags. Flavors not used within 12 months should be rejected. Each flavor should be properly codified and given an identification number.

Tips in Flavoring

The final selection of flavor for a pharmaceutical product has to be a highly subjective decision. However, some facts may well be remembered in this respect. The aldehydes in general have a pleasing flavor and can be gainfully employed for flavoring of products for internal use. The benzaldehyde and cinnamic aldehyde are too well known for their desirable odorific qualities. Acetaldehyde has a sherry-like odor. Citral is lime like. Similarly, aldehydes in oil of orange are responsible for its top note.

Phenols as class give a numbing sensation in the mouth and can be used to mask highly acidic or salty taste. Thymol, eugenol, vanillin or oils of wintergreen, cloves, sassafras, cassia, etc. can be thus used. Salty taste can also be masked by anise, raspberry, etc. Chocolate flavor masks the bitter taste effectively and may prove useful in covering taste of quinine and other bitter substances.

The sharp sensations of materials like ginger and capsicum, if used judiciously, can induce saucy flavors. These flavors are particularly useful in overcoming flat and chalky taste of hydroxides of aluminium and magnesium. Peppermint and spearmint could be good adjuvants for ginger and capsicum flavors. Unpleasant odors of many drugs can be covered up with aromatic spices in conjunction with fixatives.

For substances with acrid or burning tastes acacia syrup is suitable while lemon syrup is suitable for salty or acidic compounds. Orange syrup goes well for cough syrup having acetate, bromides, citrates, etc.

These days a number of flavor enhancers or modifiers are simultaneously used. For instance, monosodium glutamate is considered to be a potential flavor modifier for pharmaceutical preparation. Other commonly used flavor modifier is vanillin. The flavor modifiers often overcome unpleasant tastes making over flavoring unnecessary.

A survey of commonly used flavors in commercial propriety medicines has indicated that most commonly used flavors are cherry, orange, raspberry, chocolate mint and anise. Other less favored flavors are grape, black currant, strawberry, lime, tangerine, apricot, banana and pineapple.

SWEETENING AGENTS

Taste

Taste is one of the five special senses, in humans and other animals, by which four gustatory qualities (sweetness, sourness, saltiness, and bitterness) of a substance are distinguished. Taste is determined by receptors, called taste buds, the number and shape of which may vary greatly between one person and another. In general, women have more taste buds than men. A greater number of taste buds appear to endow a greater sensitivity to sweetness, sourness, saltiness, and bitterness. In humans, the taste buds are located on the surface and sides of the tongue, the roof of the mouth, and the entrance to the pharynx. The mucous membrane lining these areas is invested with tiny projections of papillae, each of which, in turn, is invested with 200 to 300 taste buds (Fig. 2.1). The papillae located at the back of the tongue, and called circumvallate, are arranged to form a V with the angle pointing backward; they transmit the sensation of bitterness.

Those at the tip of the tongue transmit sweetness, whereas saltiness and sourness are transmitted from the papillae on the sides of the tongue. Each flask-shaped taste bud contains an opening at its base through which nerve fibers enter. These

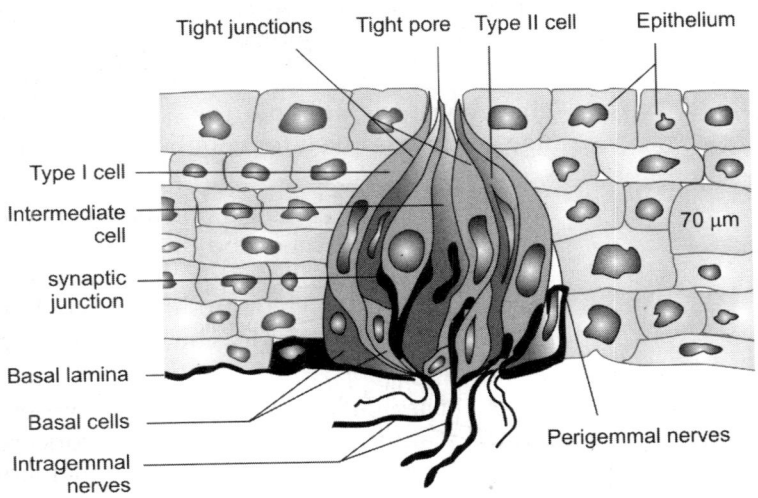

Fig. 2.1: Taste buds and its associated structures

fibers transmit impulses directly to the brain. In order for a substance to stimulate these impulses, however, it must be in solution, moistened by the salivary glands. Sensations of taste have been determined to be strongly interrelated with sensations of smell (Figs 2.1 and 2.2).

Taste is again a chemical sense and its appreciation results from the contract between the taste processing material and the 9000 taste buds in the oral cavity. Four primary tastes, viz. sweet, bitter, sour and saline are recognized and all other tastes are considered to be admixtures of one or more fundamental tastes in varying degrees. Tastes are also sometimes considered to be mixed perception involving flavors and sounds, etc. Adjustment of taste is considered essential for oral preparations. A survey of the taste preferences of the human race, as a whole, indicates sweet taste is agreeable to our species and almost

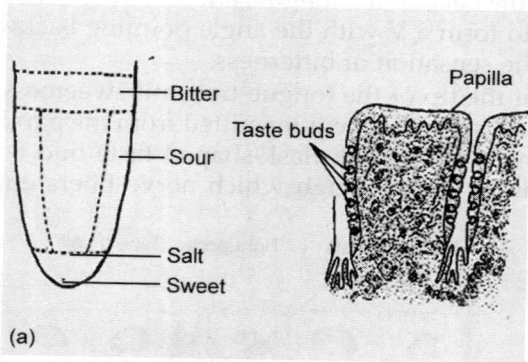

(a)

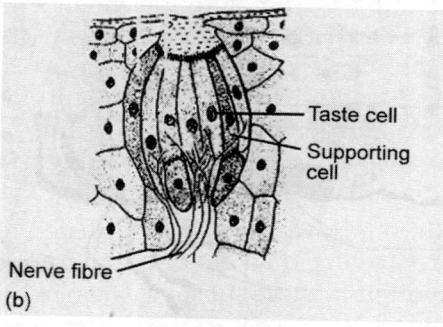

(b)

Fig. 2.2: Taste receptors and cross sectional view of taste bud

every human being accepts this taste without reservations. Hence, for controlling the taste qualities efforts have been directed towards making the preparations sweet to different degrees.

Taste Buds

There are several thousand taste buds, which you can see on your tongue. Taste buds are actually tiny nerve endings that allow us to perceive different tastes, including:

- **Salty** (i.e. French fries, peanuts)
- **Sweet** (i.e. cotton candy, strawberries)
- **Sour** (i.e. shock tarts, lemons)
- **Bitter** (i.e. black licorice, radishes)
- **Umami** (a specific taste in meat)

These nerve endings transmit messages directly to the brain by **chemical reactions.**

Sugars such as cane sugar, glucose with or without complimentary compounds like sorbitol, glycerin, etc. have been used as sweetening agents from the very beginning. Sugar coating of pills was an ancient technique and simple syrup has been used as vehicle for many oral preparations. Sugars often comprise the appreciable portions of solid dosage forms such as tablets. Cane sugar is stable between pH 4 to 8 and is generally used along with glycerin or sorbitol which reduces its tendency to get crystallized. Liquid glucose, prepared by partial hydrolysis of starch is also very suitable for sweetening of liquid preparations. Although the chemical composition of liquid glucose is not precise like molasses or the honey yet it has posed no problems. However, the chief draw back with all sugars is their liability to microbial growths. Further, sugars such as lactose and maltose have very limited sweetening power and as such the same are required to be used in larger amounts (Table 2.3).

Amongst the other sweetening agents listed above saccharin and cyclamates have had an era of popularity chiefly because very small amounts of these substances can make formulations appreciably sweet. Saccharin has a structural formula as below and can be easily synthesized starting with toluene.

Table 2.3: Sweetening agents

Sweetening agent	Relative sweetness compared to sucrose
a. L-Aspartyl-1-phenylalanine	250
b. Cyclamate	40
c. Dextrose	0.75
d. D-Fructose	1.73
e. Glycerrhizin	50
f. Lactose	0.16
g. Maltose	0.32
h. Mannitol	0.6
i. Neohesperidin dihydrochalcone	2,000
j. Saccharin	450
k. Sorbitol	0.5
l. Sucrose	1
m. Xylitol	1

Saccharin is also marketed as saccharin or saccharin sodium in which the hydrogen group in NH group is replaced by Na and which in crystalline form also has two molecules of water crystallization. Sodium saccharin can easily prepared by dissolving saccharin in equimolecular quantities of sodium hydroxide solution followed by crystallization. Sodium saccharin is nearly 200 times more soluble in water in comparison to saccharin. Saccharin is reputed to be nearly 450 times sweeter than sucrose in dilute solutions. Cyclamates are the sodium or potassium salts of cyclohexene sulfuric acid.

Previously National Formulary of USA included monographs on solutions and tablets containing sodium cyclamate and sodium saccharin. The solution contained 60% of sodium cyclamate and 6% of sodium saccharin and sweetening power of 1 ml of this solution was reckoned to be equal to 4.8 gm of sucrose. Tablets used to contain 50 mg of sodium cyclamate and 5 mg of sodium saccharin and one tablet had a sweetening power equivalent to 4 gm of sucrose.

Both saccharin and the cyclamates have been very popular with the pharmaceutical and food manufacturers. At one time these compounds were considered to be absolutely safe but some recent reports have turned the tables against them. Some countries have banned the use of these compounds while some others in process of doing so because they are found to be carcinogenic. Hence, before including these sweeteners in a preparation the manufacturer should check up the law regarding their use.

COSOLVENT

The solubility of a weak electrolyte or non-polar compound in water can be improved by changing the polarity of the solvent. This can be achieved by the addition of another solvent that is both miscible with water and in which the compound is also soluble. This process is known as cosolvency, and the solvents used in combination to increase the solubility of the solute are known as cosolvents vehicles used in combination to increase the solubility of a drug are called cosolvents, and often the solubility in this mixed system is greater than can be predicted from the materials solubility in each individual solvent.

Because it has been shown that the solubility of a given drug is maximal at a particular dielectric constant of any solvent system, it is possible to eliminate those solvent blends possessing other dielectric constants. The choice of suitable cosolvents is somewhat limited for pharmaceutical use because of possible toxicity and irritancy, particularly if required for oral or parenteral use. Ideally, suitable blends should possess values of dielectric constant between 25 and 80. The most widely used system that will cover this range is a water/ethanol mixture. Other suitable solvents for use with water include sorbitol, glycerol, propylene glycol and syrup. For example, a mixture of propylene glycol and water is used to improve the solubility of co-trimoxazole, and paracetamol is formulated as an elixir by the use of alcohol, propylene glycol and syrup. For external application to the scalp, betamethasone valerate is available dissolved in water/isopropyl alcohol mixture.

Mechanism of Cosolvency

The mechanism responsible for solubility enhancement through cosolvency is not clearly understood. It is believed that a cosolvent system works by reducing the interfacial tension between the predominately aqueous solutions and the hydrophobic solute. Recent work supports the theory that amides absorb to the solute at the interface with water, thereby diminishing the hydrophobic surface or solute/water interfacial tension. As a result, the soluble hydrophilic portion of the amide cosolvent remains oriented towards the aqueous phase.

Ethanol, sorbitol, glycerin, propylene glycol, and several members of the polyethylene glycol polymer series represent the limited number of cosolvents that are both useful and generally acceptable in the formulation of aqueous liquids. In non-aqueous solvents used in parenteral products there are a number of solvents that might also be useful in oral liquids. These include glycerol dimethylketal, N-(β-hydroxyethyl)-lactamide, ethyl lactate, ethyl carbonate, and 1,3-butylene glycol. It should be emphasized, however, that with the possible exception of dimethylacetamide, all of these solvents are unproven with respect to their acceptability for systemic use. Dimethylacetamide has been used as a cosolvent in parenteral products, but its use in oral liquids is seriously limited; owing to the difficulty of masking its objectionable odor and taste.

Application of Cosolvents

Cosolvents are employed not only to effect solubility of the drug, but also to improve the solubility of volatile constituents used to impart a desired flavor and odor to the product.

In a paint stripping formulation, the main ingredient is the active solvent able to diffuse in the reticulated film and to break the adhesive bonds between film and substrate.

Figure 2.3 shows behaviour of polar solvent
   a. In absence of co-solvent
   b. In presence of co-solvent

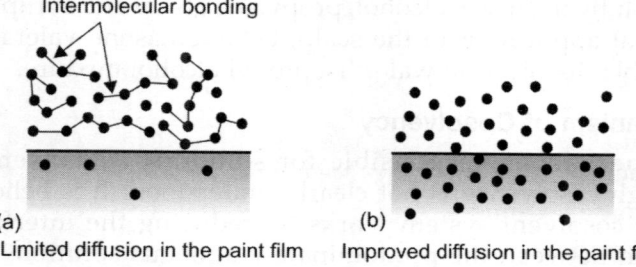

Intermolecular bonding

(a)   (b)

Limited diffusion in the paint film   Improved diffusion in the paint film

Fig. 2.3: Showing behavior of a polar solvent

DMSO (cosolvent) is a choice solvent to formulate efficient paint stripper. The addition of other components in the paint stripping formulation will help to adjust performances: When formulating **DMSO-based paint stripper**, the following family of co-solvents can be used: Ketones (methylethylketone —MEK, methylisobutylketone—MIBK, ethylamylketone—AK, etc.), ethers, esthers and green solvents.

PRESERVATIVES

A **preservative** is a natural or synthetic chemical that is added to products such as foods, pharmaceuticals, paints, biological samples, wood, etc. to prevent decomposition by microbial growth or by undesirable chemical changes. All of these chemicals act as either antimicrobials or antioxidants or both. They either inhibit the activity of or kill the bacteria, molds, insects and other microorganisms. Antimicrobials, prevent the growth of molds, yeasts and bacteria and antioxidants keep foods from becoming rancid or developing black spots. They suppress the reaction when foods comes in contact with oxygen, heat, and some metals. They also prevent the loss of some essential amino acids and some vitamins. Majority of pharmaceutical formulations are liable to microbial growth, which may lead by large scale chemical changes even otherwise presence of microbial flora in any pharmaceutical preparation is against normal principles of hygiene. Hence, all pharmaceutical preparations, which are capable of supporting microbial metabolism, and which are to be stored over appreciable periods of time, have to be properly preserved. Further potential products packed in multidose vials are necessarily required to carry such an amount of an antimicrobial compound which can serve doses. Only a few compounds like phenol, chlorocresol, phenyl mercuric nitrate, etc. have been cleared by the pharmacopoeias in this respect. Preservation of products is ensured by inclusion of right proportions of suitable antiseptics. The most commonly employed antiseptics for pharmaceutical formulations are (Table 2.4):

- Benzoic acid and benzoates
- Boric acid
- Chlorobenzoic acid (ortho and para)

Table 2.4: Some common preservatives and their primary activity

Chemical affected	Organism(s)	Action	Use in foods
Sulfites	Insects and microorganisms	Antioxidant	Dried fruits, wine, juice
Sodium nitrite	Clostridia	Antimicrobial	Cured meats
Propionic acid	Molds	Antimicrobial	Bread, cakes, cheeses
Sorbic acid	Molds	Antimicrobial	Cheeses, cakes, salad
Benzoic acid	Yeasts and molds	Antimicrobial	Soft drinks, ketchup

- Dehydroacetic acid
- Formic acid and formaldehyde
- Parachlorometacresol
- Parachlorometaxylenol
- Parahydroxybenzoates (parabens)
- Phenylhexachlorophen
- Phenylmercuric acid
- Propionic acid
- Quaternary ammonium compounds like benzalkonium chloride, cetrimide, etc.
- Salicylic acid and salicylates
- 2, 2-thio-bis 4, 6-dichlorophenol (actamer)
- 3, 4, 4-trichlorosalicylanilide (anobial).

Benzoic acid and benzoates: Benzoic acid is used as a preservative for food, drugs, cosmetics, etc. either as such or in the form of sodium and potassium benzoate. It is generally used in concentration of 0.1%.

Salicylic acid and salicylates: Salicylic acid is generally used as sodium salicylate to the extent of 1 part in 1000.

Parahydroxybenzoates (parabens): Various esters of p-hydroxybenzoic acid having methyl, ethyl, propyl, and butyl radicals are marketed by different firms under names such as 'Nipa' series 'parabens', etc. Different esters have diffent solubility in organic solvents. Their solubility in water are generally low but sodium salts dissolve freely. The 'preservative' concentrations of these compounds are low ranging from 0.005 to 0.05. These esters are considered to be 2 to 3 times as effective as benzoic acid and higher the alkyl group in the ester more powerful is the preservative.

Phenyl mercuric nitrate and other salts: These compounds are used for cosmetics at concentrations not exceeding 0.01%, and are also recognized preservatives of pharmaceutical products for parenteral use. Phenyl mercuric nitrate is included in multiple dose packing of parenteral products and in preparations which are sterilized by 'heating with bactericide.

Parachlorometacresol: This compound is also recommended for inclusion in multiple dose vials of parenteral products and for sterilization by 'heating with bactericide'. Most preparations are preserved by including 0.1% of this compound. Its use in food products is, however banned.

Parachlorometaxylenol: It is an important antiseptic and solutions containing up to 0.5% are employed as antiseptics for cuts and wounds and in surgical. It may be used as preservative for preparations which are meant for external use. About 1% concentration is used for these purposes.

Phenol: It is used in lotions and other preparations meant for external use. It can also be used in parenteral products packed as multiple doses in concentrations of 0.5%. Several pharmacopoeias recognize it as antiseptic or sterilizaton by 'heating with bactericide' method, the recommended concentration being 0.5%.

Actamer: Actamer is a colorless, odourless, powder soluble to the extent of 0.0004% in water. The solubility increases appreciably of addition of sodium hydroxide due to formation of sodium salts. It is employed as an ingredient of soaps and skin cosmetics. It is effective against fungi and bacteria.

Anobial: Anobial is a yellowish grey powder having phenolic odour and dissolving to the extent of 0.0015% in water. It is used as an ingredient of soaps and is effective in the control of skin flora.

Quaternary ammonium compounds: Many quaternary compounds have come up as useful antimicrobial compound notable being benzalkonium chloride, cetyl trimethylammonium bromide, etc. These compounds are effective in low concentrations but are inactivated by anionic material such as soaps, lauryl sulfate, cetyl sulfate, etc.

Formaldehyde: Formaldehyde continues to be a good preservative for different kinds of material though its use for pharmaceutical products is almost nil. It has strong pungent and irritant properties and not a good preservative.

Desirable Characteristics of Preservatives

The preservatives should have following characteristics:

1. Must be able to stop growth of very wide range of microbes.
2. Must be chemically compatible with other ingredients of the formulation and should remain 'intact' during the life time of the dosage form.
3. Must be non-toxic and non-sensitizing.
4. Should dissolve in adequate proportions in the aqueous phase.

Natural Food Preservatives

Natural substances such as salt, sugar, vinegar, and diatomaceous earth are also used as traditional preservatives. Certain processes such as freezing, pickling, smoking and salting can also be used to preserve food. Another group of preservatives targets enzymes in fruits and vegetables that continue to metabolize after they are cut. For instance, citric and ascorbic acids from lemon or other citrus juice can inhibit the action of the enzyme phenolase which turns surfaces of cut apples and potatoes brown. Caution must be taken, however, since FDA standards do not currently require fruit and vegetable product labels to accurately reflect the type of preservative used in the products.

Uses

No single antimicrobial compound possesses all the above mentioned qualities. Nowadays combination of two or more preservatives is used for broader spectrum of antimicrobial activity. In selective a preservative its effect on pH of the product must also be kept in mind. Some of the commonly used compounds such as phenol chlorocresol, esters of benzoic and p-hydroxybenzoic acid, etc. are acidic in nature while compounds like chlorobutanol phenylethyl alcohol, etc. are neutral.

For a large category of pharmaceutical formulation for oral use, the preservatives are generally drawn from the acidic group parahydroxybenzoates being the most popular. For ophthalmic, nasal or parenteral products, the mercurials, quaternary ammonium compounds, as well as neutral preservatives are more preferred. However, many mercurial compounds are readily reduced to mercury which quaternary compounds are inactivated by anionic substances.

SURFACTANTS

Interface

The behavior of molecules situated at or near the boundary between two immiscible liquids phases like oil and water is called interface. In the body of matter the molecules experience equal attraction in all directions and as such, no resultant forces act on any molecule. At the interface the molecule is pulled by similar molecules in some directions and by dissimilar molecules in some other direction. Since the forces between like molecules are of a greater magnitude than the forces between the unlike molecules, molecules at the interface have a tendency to leave the interface and reduce the area of contact. Bringing in of more molecules is consequently resisted and the interface behaves as if it is under tension in a tangential direction. The magnitude of this tension per unit length is called interfacial tension. In air-liquid interface the force is referred to as the surface tension. The value of interfacial tension depends primarily upon the chemical nature of the molecules and to some extent on the temperature, since change in temperature brings about change in the thermal energy of the molecules. In pharmaceutical systems, which are often heterogeneous, many problems arise because of interfacial tension between the different phases. These types of problems can be handled by proper selection of surfactants.

Surfactant

Surfactants are materials which have a tendency to pre-ferentially get absorbed at the interface between two phases.

Their molecules consist of a *'polar'* and a *'non-polar'* part and when they are placed between two phases of differing polarities the non-polar part gets oriented towards the phase of low polarity while the polar towards the high polarity phase. As a result of their surface absorption the tension between two phases gets lowered and the phases acquire a greater tendency to intermix with each other. Hence, wherever there is need to lower the interfacial tension surfactants are used.

When a surfactant is placed in a solvent, its molecules are present in a larger number at the interface than in the bulk of the solution. Preferential absorption at the interface continues until all the available space at the surface is occupied. Thereafter the surfactants molecules descend into the bulk of the solution in the form of molecular aggregates or micelles of various shapes. The molecules are so arranged in a micelle that their parts, corresponding to polarity of the solution, are oriented towards the outside. The concentration of the surfactant at which it forms micelle is known as *critical micelle concentration* (*CMC*). Figure 2.4 illustrates the surface adsorption of surfactants and micelle formation.

Structure of Surfactants Molecules

The surfactants molecules consist both of polar and non-polar parts. The polarity and non-polarity are due to various radicals and groups. Some groups possessing polar and non-polar qualities are listed in Table 2.5.

Table 2.5: List of polar and non-polar groups

Polar groups	Non-polar groups
Aldehyde	Alcohols (higher)
Amino	Alkyl groups 8–18 carbon atoms
Carboxyl	Alkyl groups 3–8 carbon atoms
Ether	Benzene
Ketone	Naphthalene
Metallic salts sulfonate	Polyoxypropylene
Nitro	Rosin acids
Phosphates	Terpenes
Polyoxyethylene	Hydrocarbons 8–20 carbon atoms or more
Sulfonic acid	Olefins (mono) 8–20 carbon atoms or more

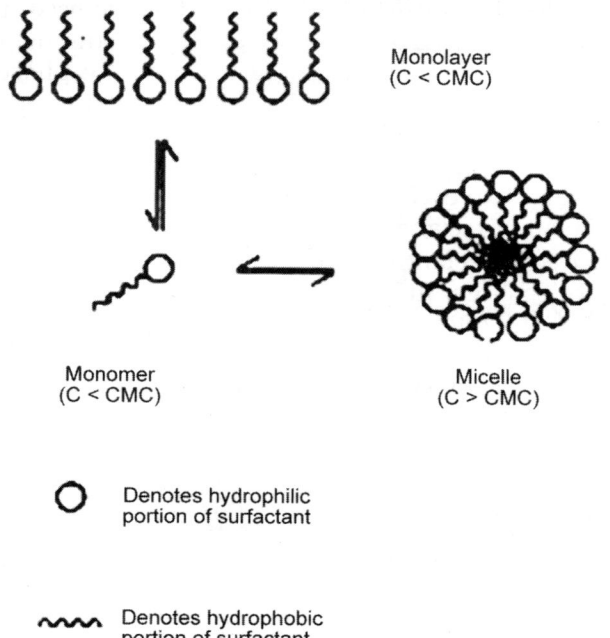

Monolayer
(C < CMC)

Monomer
(C < CMC)

Micelle
(C > CMC)

O   Denotes hydrophilic
     portion of surfactant

~~~ Denotes hydrophobic
     portion of surfactant

Fig. 2.4: Surface absorption of surfactants and micelle formation

If these groups are linked together either directly or through an ester, ether and acid amide linkage surfactant molecules are produced.

The behavior of a given surfactant in a solution would largely be governed by relative magnitude of the hydrophilic and hydrophobic groups constituting it. If the hydrophilic group is stronger compound it is ready to dissolve in water or other polar solvents since polar groups will overcome the tendency of non-polar groups to resist dissolution. Similarly, if the hydrophobic groups be more powerful it will not allow the surfactant to dissolve in water but will tend to drag the molecule in non-polar phase. If the relative proportion of the hydrophobic and hydrophilic groups are balanced the molecule will have appreciable tendency to orient at the interface.

Figure 2.5 represents different balances of non-polar and polar groups.

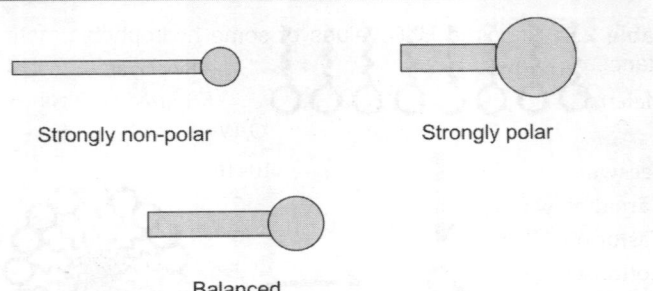

Strongly non-polar   Strongly polar

Balanced

Fig. 2.5: Types of balances of polar and non-polar groups

Evaluation of Hydrophobic and Hydrophilic Parts of Surfactant

Griffin devised a method HLB system and was based on the balance between the hydrophilic and hydrophobic portions of the surfactant molecules. Each surfactant was assigned a number known as its HLB value which ranged from 1 to 40. Increase in the number of the HLB value was indicative of simultaneous increase in the hydrophilic properties of the surfactant (Table 2.6).

For many non-ionic surfactants HLB values can be calculated by use of simple equation developed by Griffin. It is deemed to be percentage weight of hydrophilic groups divided by 5 in order to reduce the range of the HLB values. As such a 100% hydrophilic molecule like polyethylene glycol will have a HLB value of 20. This can be generalized by the following equation:

$$HLB = E/5$$

where, E is the weight percentage of the hydrophilic groups. In case a molecule has other hydrophilic groups like polyhydric alcohols the HLB values can be calculated by the following equation:

$$HLB = E + P/5$$

where, P is the weight percentage of the polyhydric alcohols and E that of the polyoxyethylene groups. The HLB values of fatty esters of polyhydric alcohol such as spans can be calculated by the following equation:

$$HLB = 20(1-S/A)$$

Table 2.6: Required HLB values of some hydrophobic material substances

Material	Required HLB values	
	O/W	W/O
Beeswax	10–16	5
Carnauba wax	12	–
Castor oil	14	–
Cottonseed oil	7.5	–
Cetyl alcohol	13	–
Lanolin (anhydrous)	15	8
Lauryl alcohol	14	–
Lauric acid	15–16	–
Methyl silicone	11	–
Mineral oil (light)	10–12	4
Mineral oil (heavy)	10.5	4
Oleic acid	17	–
Paraffin wax	9	–
Petrolatum	7–8	–
Stearic acid	17	–

Here S and A are the saponification and acid numbers of the fatty acid.

Davies suggested another approach for the calculation of the HLB values based on a concept that hydrophilic groups make a positive and hydrophobic group a negative contribution to the HLB values. He assigned values to various hydrophilic and hydrophobic groups and called them "group *numbers*". If the molecular structure of a surfactant is known the groups numbers can be substituted in the following equation in order to calculate the HLB values:

$$\text{HLB} = \Sigma \, (\text{hydrophilic group number}) - (\text{group number of} - CH_2 \text{ group}) + 7$$

Classification

A surfactant can be classified by the presence of formally charged groups in its head. A non-ionic surfactant has no charge groups in its head. The head of an ionic surfactant carries a net charge. If the charge is negative, the surfactant is more

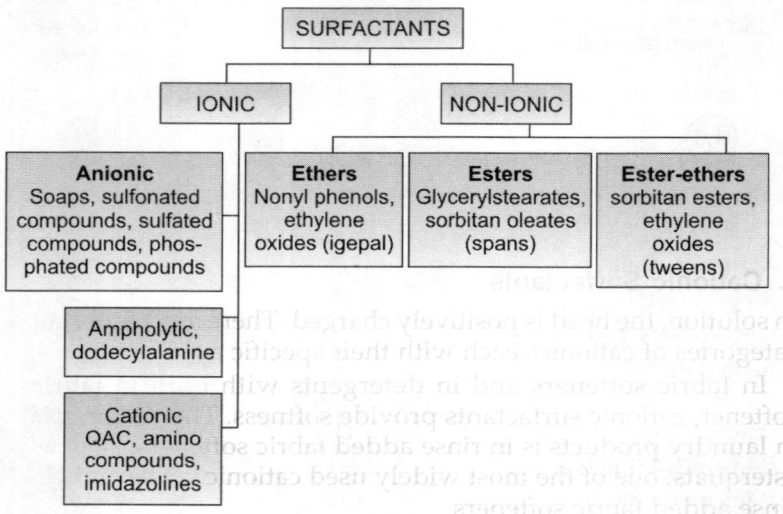

specifically called anionic; if the charge is positive, it is called cationic. If a surfactant contains a head with two oppositely charged groups, it is termed **zwitter ion.** Some commonly encountered surfactants of each type include the following:

1. Anionic Surfactants

In solution, the head is negatively charged. This is the most widely used type of surfactant for laundering, dishwashing liquids and shampoos because of its excellent cleaning properties and high. The surfactant is particularly good at keeping the dirt away from fabrics, and removing residues of fabric softener from fabrics. Anionic surfactants are particularly effective at oily soil cleaning and oil/clay soil suspension. Still, they can react in the wash water with the positively charged water hardness ions (calcium and magnesium), which can lead to partial deactivation. The more calcium and magnesium molecules in the water, the more the anionic surfactant system suffers from deactivation. To prevent this, the anionic surfactants need help from other ingredients such as builders (Ca/Mg sequestrants) and more detergent should be dosed in hard water.

The most commonly used anionic surfactants are alkyl sulphates, alkyl ethoxylate sulphates and soaps.

Linear alkyl sulfate

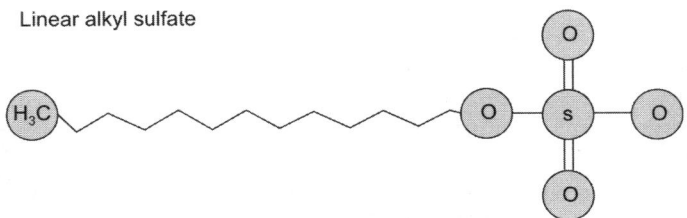

2. Cationic Surfactants

In solution, the head is positively charged. There are 3 different categories of cationics each with their specific application.

In fabric softeners and in detergents with built-in fabric softener, cationic surfactants provide softness. Their main use in laundry products is in rinse added fabric softeners, such as esterquats, one of the most widely used cationic surfactants in rinse added fabric softeners.

An example of cationic surfactants is the monoalkyl quaternary system

Monoalkyl quaternary system

3. Non-ionic Surfactants

These surfactants do not have an electrical charge, which makes them resistant to water hardness deactivation. They are excellent grease removers that are used in laundry products, household cleaners and hand dishwashing liquids.

Most laundry detergents contain both non-ionic and anionic surfactants as they complement each other's cleaning action. Non-ionic surfactants contribute to making the surfactant system less hardness sensitive. The most commonly used non-ionic surfactants are ethers of fatty alcohols.

Non-ionic surfactants

4. Amphoteric/Zwitterionic Surfactant

These surfactants are very mild, making them particularly suited for use in personal care and household cleaning products. They can be anionic (negatively charged), cationic (positively charged) or non-ionic (no charge) in solution, depending on the acidity or pH of the water.

They are compatible with all other classes of surfactants and are soluble and effective in the presence of high concentrations of electrolytes, acids and alkalis.

These surfactants may contain two charged groups of different sign. Whereas the positive charge is almost always ammonium, the source of the negative charge may vary (carboxylate, sulphate, sulphonate). These surfactants have excellent dermatological properties. They are frequently used in shampoos and other cosmetic products, and also in hand dishwashing liquids because of their high foaming properties. An example of an amphoteric/zwitterionic surfactant is alkyl betaine.

Alkyl betaine

5. Difference Between Anionic and Nonionic Surfactants

Surfactant is a substance which has both a hydrophilic group and a hydrophobic group. Concerning the name, a surfactant which dissociates in water and releases cation and anion (or zwitterions) is termed ionic (cationic, anionic, zwitterionic) surfactant. On the other hand, a surfactant which does not dissociate is called a nonionic surfactant.

An anionic surfactant has an anionic hydrophilic group. Examples of anionic surfactants are generally called "soap" (fatty acid soap), alkylsulfonic acid salts (the main component of synthetic detergent, such as linear alkyl benzene sulfonate (LAS), fatty alcohol sulfate (the main component of shampoo or old neutral detergents), etc.

Because fatty acid soap is a salt of fatty acid and alkali metal (a salt of a weak acid and a strong base), it hydrolyzes in water and the solution becomes slightly basic. However, the solutions of other anionic surfactants are neutral. The solution of synthetic detergent is adjusted to slightly basic, but this is not because of the detergent itself (it is neutral) but because of the effect of auxiliary agents (sodium carbonate, etc). This is the main difference between soap and synthetic detergent.

Animal fibers, such as silk and wool, are called "amphoteric fibers", which means that the fibers can become both cationic and anionic, depending on the property of the liquid. If alkaline detergents (both powder soap and synthetic detergent) are used for washing these fibers, anionic surfactant would adsorb on the cationic groups (amino groups) on the fiber. It would be possible to wash poor alkali-proof fiber by maintaining a neutral pH. However, we cannot do anything about the ionic adsorption of surfactant on fibers. This is one of the advantages of non-ionic surfactants. There is a detergent that can wash clothes which have the "dry cleaning sign" (the picture sign for recommending that dry cleaning be done, found on silk and wool products) by water at home. As you may already realize, the main component of this type of detergent is non-ionic surfactant. Since electrostatic force does not work for non-ionic surfactants, the amount of detergent remaining after washing would be low for other kinds of clothes as well as for silk and wool.

There is a possibility that anionic surfactants combine with cationic ions, for example, calcium ion in hard water. Especially in the case of powder soaps, fatty acids combine with calcium ions and form scum, which is not water-soluble and precipitates, decreasing the cleaning effect. Other anionic surfactants also combine with calcium, but these amounts would be low. Anyway, no precipitation happens if non-ionic surfactant is used. So this point is also one of the advantages of non-ionic surfactants.

Application

Surfactants also have an important role in our body, where they are used to reduce surface tension in the lungs. The human body does not start to produce lung surfactants until late in foetal development. Therefore, premature babies are often unable to breathe properly, a condition called respiratory distress syndrome if untreated, this is a serious illness and is often fatal, but administration of artificial surfactants virtually eliminates this health problem.

Hydrophilic lipophilic balance (HLB) of a surfactant was devised by Griffin (Fig. 2.6 and Table 2.7).

$$HLB = 20\,(1\text{-saponification value/acid value})$$

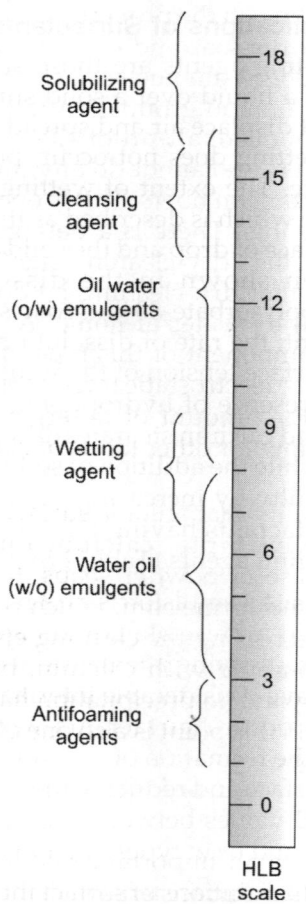

Fig. 2.6: HLB scale

Table 2.7: HLB value of some common agents

HLB value	Agents
1–3	Antifoaming agents
3–7	Ariacell
3–8	Water/oil emulgents
7–9	Wetting and spreading agents
8–16	Oil/water emulgents
16–40	Solubilizing agents

Pharmaceutical Applications of Surfactants

Wetting agents: Wetting agents are those substances which helps in spreading of a liquid over a solid surface. For this to occur, the liquid must displace air and spread over the surface of the solid. If the wetting does not occur, powder will float and tend to aggregate. The extent of wetting is measured in terms of contact angle which is described as the angle between the tangent to the surface of drop and the solid surface. Marked increases have been shown in the dissolution rate of Phenobarbital when polysorbate-80 is used in simulated gastric fluids as wetting agent; the rate of dissolution is proportional to the reduction in surface tension of the solution. Similarly in case of tablets, the presence of hydrophobic tablet lubricants such as magnesium and calcium stearates decreases dissolution rate of salicylic acid while the addition of sodium lauryl sulfate overcomes this difficulty by increasing the wettability of the tablet. Generally surfactants having HLB values in between 7 and 9 are good wetting agents (Table 2.8).

Emulsifying agents: An emulsion is a biphasic liquid dosage form in which the two immiscible liquids are made miscible with the help of an emulsifying agent. The water and oil (two immiscible phases) have considerable interfacial tension and a dispersion does not occur. Surfactants which are used as emulsifiers facilitate the formation of an emulsion by orienting themselves at the interface and reducing the interfacial tension. Surfactants with HLB values between 3–8 and 9–16 promote the formation of o/w and o/w types of emulsion respectively.

Solubilizing agents: Solutions of surfactants have the ability to dissolve substances which are insoluble by reducing the

Table 2.8: The HLB values of some common surfactants

Compound	HLB value
Sodium lauryl sulfate	40.0
Sodium oleate	18.0
Polyoxyethylene monostearate (Myrj 52)	16.9
Polyoxyethylene lauryl ether (Brij 35)	16.9
Polyoxyethylene sorbitan monolaurate (Tween-20)	16.7
Polyoxyethylene sorbitan monopalmitate (Tween-40)	15.6
Polyoxyethylene sorbitan monooleate (Tween-80)	15.0
Polyoxyethylene castor oil	13.3
Polyoxyethylene sorbitan monolaurate (Tween-21)	13.3
Tragacanth	13.2
Triethanolamine oleate (Trolamine)	12.0
Gelatin	9.8
Sorbitan monolaurate (Span 20)	8.6
Sorbitan monopalmitate (Span-40)	6.7
Glyceryl monostearate (Aldo 28)	5.5
Sorbitan monostearate (Ariacel 60)	4.7
Sorbitan monooleate (Span-80)	4.3
Sorbitan tristearate (Span-65)	2.1
Sorbitan trioleate (Span-85)	1.8

interfacial tension between them. Drugs having low aqueous solubility have been solubilized by using solubilizing agents. Examples are oil soluble vitamins, steroid hormones and antimicrobial agents. The fundamental process involves the use of a surfactant which forms micelles in water consisting of 100 to 150 molecules. The order of these aggregations is such that in water phase the hydrophobic groups of the molecules are oriented towards the center while the polar parts face the water. In order to act as good solubilizing agents surfactants should have HLB values between 16 and 19.

Foaming and antifoaming agents: Foams are generally needed in some cosmetic preparations. Foaming agents promote the formation of stable foams. Foams are emulsions of gases in liquids and need some surfactant(s) for physical stability.

Antifoaming agents are those substances which prevents foam formation, in many pharmaceutical formulation foaming is not desired because it causes difficulty in measuring the exact amount needed for dispensing. Generally substances with HLB values between 1 and 3 are good antifoaming agents. In pharmaceutical formulations, alcohol and silicones are normally employed as antifoaming agents.

ANTIOXIDANTS

The active drug present in a formulation should not get degraded during its shelf life. Even very minor changes in their chemical configuration could result in drastic changes in their pharmacologic actions. Amongst the many changes brought about by environmental factors, oxidation of drug molecules is the most serious change. An antioxidant is a **molecule** capable of slowing or preventing the **oxidation** of other molecules. Oxidation is a **chemical reaction** that transfers **electrons** from a substance to an **oxidizing agent.** Oxidation reactions can produce **free radicals,** which start **chain reactions** that damage **cells.** Antioxidants terminate these chain reactions by removing free radical intermediates, and inhibit other oxidation reactions by being oxidized themselves. Hence, antioxidants are often **reducing agents.** Some drugs which undergo oxidation are given in Table 2.9.

Table 2.9: Commonly used drugs sensitive to oxidation

Amikacin	Kanamycin
Ascorbic acid	Metoclopramide
Chlorpromazine	Morphine
Cyanocobalamin	Neomycin
Dexamethasone	Norepinephrine
Hydrocortisone	Novobiocin
Reserpine	Paraldehyde
Resorcinol	Penicillin
Riboflavine	Tetracyclines
Streptomycin	Thiamine
Prednisolone	Tobramycin
Vitamins A, D and E	Sulfadiazine

The oxidation is either addition of oxygen or withdrawal of hydrogen or of from a chemical molecule. Every time a molecule is oxidized another molecule simultaneously gets reduced. Antioxidants are added in the formulation of drugs which are liable to oxidative degradation. The antioxidants may by categorized as:

1. True antioxidants which act by breaking the free radical chain.
2. Synergist which generally act by enhancing the action of true antioxidants.

Antioxidants are widely distributed in nature and occur in many plants and as components of fats and oils, among the natural antioxidants the tocopherols are the most widely distributed ones. A large number of antioxidants, both inorganic and organic have been developed in laboratories. Antioxidants are classified into two broad divisions, depending on whether they are soluble in water (hydrophilic) or in lipids (hydrophobic). In general, water-soluble antioxidants react with oxidants in the cell cytosol and the blood plasma, while lipid-soluble antioxidants protect cell membranes from lipid peroxidation. These compounds may be synthesized in the body or obtained from the diet. Some of the modern antioxidants used in foods, drugs and cosmetics are discussed in the following sections.

Water Soluble Antioxidants

The main classes of water soluble antioxidants are sulfurous acid salts, ascorbic acid isomers and thiol derivatives. The important characteristics storage requirements and uses of compounds of this class are given in Table 2.10.

Oil Soluble Antioxidants

The oil soluble antioxidants are often needed for the protection of fatty foods and cosmetics. In the pharmaceutical field formulations like ointments, oily injections, etc. containing oxygen sensitive drugs may require protection by antioxidants. Table 2.11 lists the important oil soluble antioxidants.

BHA 2% is generally used as a mixture with propyl gallate 6%, citric acid 4% and propylene glycol 70% chiefly for foods and cosmetics. This can also prevent oxidation of fats at concentrations of 0.02%. BHT is used for vegetable oils and

Table 2.10: Compounds their pH, concentration required and storage conditions

Compound	pH	Drugs	Concentration	Storage
Sodium bisulfite	Acidic	Steroids, antibiotics adrenergics, and morphine	0.05%	Away from light. Below 40°C in a air tight container
Sodium metabisulfite	Acidic	Epinephrine	0.025 to 0.1%	Away from light. Below 40°C in a air tight container
Sodium sulfite	Alkaline	Reserpine chlor-promazine	0.01 to 0.2%	Away from light. Below 40°C in a air tight container
Sodium formaldehyde sulfoxylate	Alkaline	Procaine penicillin	0.005 to 0.15%	Away from light. Below 40°C in a air tight container
Sodium thiosulfate	Alkaline	Sodium, sulfac-etamide	0.1–0.5%	Away from light. Below 40°C in a air tight container
L-Ascorbic acid	Acidic	Epinephrine, ferrous sulfate	0.2–0.5%	Away from light. Below 40°C in a air tight container

Table 2.11: Compounds their uses, concentration required and storage conditions

Compound	Substances	Concentration	Storage
Ascorbyl palmitate	Foods	0.01–0.02%	Away from light. Below 40°C in a air tight container
Butylated hydroxyanisole (BHA and butylated hydroxyl toluene (BHT)	Fatty formulations	0.005–0.02%	Away from light. Below 40°C in a air tight container
Tocopherols	Vitamin E	0.05–0.75%	Away from light. Below 40°C in a air tight container

fats. It can be used to the extent of 0.01%. A combination of BHA and BHT is used for synergistic effect.

Glutathione

It is a cysteine-containing peptide found in most forms of aerobic life. It is not required in the diet and is instead synthesized in cells from its constituent amino acids. Glutathione has antioxidant properties since the thiol group in its cysteine moiety is a reducing agent and can be reversibly oxidized and reduced. In cells, glutathione is maintained in the reduced form by the enzyme glutathione reductase and in turn reduces other metabolites and enzyme systems as well as reacting directly with oxidants. Due to its high concentration and its central role in maintaining the cell's redox state, glutathione is one of the most important cellular antioxidants.

Melatonin

Melatonin is a powerful antioxidant that can easily cross cell membranes and the blood–brain barrier. Unlike other antioxidants, melatonin does not undergo redox cycling, which is the ability of a molecule to undergo repeated reduction and oxidation. Redox cycling may allow other antioxidants (such as vitamin C) to act as pro-oxidants and promote free radical formation. Melatonin, once oxidized, cannot be reduced to its former state because it forms several stable end-products upon reacting with free radicals. Therefore, it has been referred to as a terminal (or suicidal) antioxidant.

Tocopherols and Tocotrienols (Vitamin E)

Vitamin E is the collective name for a set of eight related tocopherols and tocotrienols, which are fat-soluble vitamins with antioxidant properties. Of these, α-tocopherol has been most studied as it has the highest bioavailability, with the body preferentially absorbing and metabolizing this form.

It has been claimed that the α-tocopherol form is the most important lipid-soluble antioxidant, and that it protects membranes from oxidation by reacting with lipid radicals produced in the lipid peroxidation chain reaction. This removes the free radical intermediates and prevents the propagation reaction from continuing. This reaction produces oxidized α-tocopheroxyl radicals that can be recycled back to the active reduced form through reduction by other antioxidants, such as ascorbate, retinol or ubiquinol.

However, the roles and importance of the various forms of vitamin E are presently unclear, and it has even been suggested that the most important function of α-tocopherol is as a signaling molecule, with this molecule having no significant role in antioxidant metabolism. The functions of the other forms of vitamin E are even less well-understood, although γ-tocopherol is a nucleophile that may react with electrophilic mutagens, and tocotrienols may be important in protecting neurons from damage.

Superoxide Dismutase and Catalase

Superoxide dismutases (SODs) are a class of closely related enzymes that catalyze the breakdown of the superoxide anion into oxygen and hydrogen peroxide. SOD enzymes are present in almost all aerobic cells and in extracellular fluids. Superoxide dismutase enzymes contain metal ion cofactors that, depending on the isozyme, can be copper, zinc, manganese or iron. In humans, the copper/zinc SOD is present in the cytosol, while manganese SOD is present in the mitochondrion.

Catalases are enzymes that catalyze the conversion of hydrogen peroxide to water and oxygen, using either an iron or manganese cofactor. This protein is localized to peroxisomes in most eukaryotic cells. Catalase is an unusual enzyme since, although hydrogen peroxide is its only substrate, it follows a ping-pong mechanism. Here, its cofactor is oxidized by one molecule of hydrogen peroxide and then regenerated by transferring the bound oxygen to a second molecule of substrate. Despite its apparent importance in hydrogen peroxide removal, humans with genetic deficiency of catalase—"acatalasemia" suffer a few ill effects.

Desirable Characteristics of Antioxidants

The antioxidants, must possess certain desirable qualities listed below for use in pharmaceutical preparations:

1. Must dissolve readily in the substrate.
2. Must be non-toxic and free from irritant.

3. Must by compatible with other ingredients of the formulation.

4. Should be inert

5. Only a very small quantity should be required.

6. Should be broad spectrum, i.e. act on large number of preparations.

7. Should be economical and easily available.

8. Should be able to produce the response for a long period of time.

Antioxidants are found in varying amounts in foods such as vegetables, fruits, grain cereals, legumes and nuts. Some antioxidants such as lycopene and ascorbic acid can be destroyed by long-term storage or prolonged cooking. Other antioxidant compounds are more stable, such as the polyphenolic antioxidants in foods such as whole-wheat cereals and tea. In general, processed foods contain fewer antioxidants than fresh and uncooked foods, since the preparation processes may expose the food to oxygen (Table 2.12).

Table 2.12: List of antioxidant compound and their sources

Antioxidant compounds	Foods containing antioxidants
Vitamin C (ascorbic acid)	Fruits and vegetables
Vitamin E (tocopherols, tocotrienols)	Vegetable oils
Polyphenolic antioxidants	Tea, coffee, soy, fruit, olive oil, chocolate
Carotenoids (lycopene, carotenes)	Fruit and vegetables

Some antioxidants are made in the body and are not absorbed from the intestine. One example is glutathione, which is made from amino acids. As any glutathione in the gut is broken down to free cysteine, glycine and glutamic acid before being absorbed, even large oral doses have a little effect on the concentration of glutathione in the body. Ubiquinol (coenzyme Q) is also poorly absorbed from the gut and is made in humans through the mevalonate pathway. Antioxidants are an especially important class of preservatives as, unlike bacterial or fungal spoilage, oxidation reactions still occur relatively rapidly in frozen or refrigerated food. These preservatives include ascorbic acid (AA, E300), propyl gallate (PG, E310), tocopherols (E306), tertiary butylhydroquinone (TBHQ), butylated hydroxyanisole (BHA, E320) and butylated hydroxytoluene (BHT, E321).

Uses

Antioxidants are frequently added to industrial products. Some common uses are:
- As stabilizers in fuels and lubricants to prevent oxidation
- In gasolines to prevent the polymerization that leads to the formation of engine-fouling residues.
- To prevent the oxidative degradation of polymers such as rubbers, plastics and adhesives
- As an antiozonants.
- Antioxidant preservatives are also added to fat-based cosmetics such as lipstick and moisturizers to prevent rancidity.
- Protects cells and strengthens memory
- Increases mental clarity
- Provides essential fatty acids
- Stabilizes proper cholesterol
- Scavengers for free radicals
- Builds proteins
- Strengthens nervous system, heart and cell membrane
- Fights viruses, bacteria
- Helps reduce risk of cancer
- Enhances cellular communication and strengthens immune system.

PRACTICE QUESTIONS

Q. 1. Write in brief about various pharmaceutical additives used in pharmaceutical formulation.

Q. 2. Write short notes on:
   a. Mineral colors
   b. Colors obtained from plants
   c. Colors obtained from animals.
   d. Lakes

Q. 3. What are desirable characteristics required for a coloring agent? Give various tips used in coloring?

Q. 4. What are flavouring agents? How flavouring of a pharmaceutical product is done?

Q. 5. What is the significance of matching the taste and flavour, explain it with suitable examples?

Q. 6. What are sweetening agents? Enlist various sweetening agents used for pharmaceutical formulation.

Q. 7. Write in brief about co-solvents. Give their pharmaceutical applications.

Q. 8. Define the term preservatives. Explain briefly with suitable examples their use in pharmaceutical formulations.

Q. 9. Write short notes on:
   a. Desired characteristics of preservatives
   b. Natural food preservation

Q. 10. What are surfactants? Give their classification.

Q. 11. Write short notes on:
   a. HLB value
   b. HLB scale
   c. CMC
   d. Amphoteric surfactant

Q. 12. Differentiate between cationic and anionic surfactant.

Q. 13. Give pharmaceutical application of surfactant.

Q. 14. What are antioxidants? Differentiate between water soluble and oil soluble antioxidants.

Q. 15. What are desirable characteristics of an antioxidant? Give their uses?

OBJECTIVE TYPE QUESTIONS

1. Visible radiation fall in wavelength ....

2. When all wavelengths are absorbed—then the substance will appear .... while when no wavelength is absorbed or reflected back—then the substance will appear ....

3. HLB formula for surfactant given by Griffin is ....

4. Vitamin C is .... soluble antioxidant while vitamin E is...................................... soluble antioxidant.

5. BHA and BHT are ....

6. Cochineal is a ....

7. Methyl paraben and propyl paraben are example of ....

8. HLB stands for .... , and the term HLB was given by ....

9. W/o emulgents have HLB value .... while o/w emulgents have HLB value ....

10. Match the following:

Sweetening agent	Relative sweetness
1. Aspartame	a. 450
2. Sucrose	b. 50
3. Glycerrhizin	c. 250
4. Saccharin	d. 1

11. Match the following:

HLB value	Agents
1. 1–3	a. Solubilizing agent
2. 3–7	b. Anti-foaming agent
3. 7–9	c. W/o emulgents
4. 16–40	d. Wetting agent

12. Match the following:

Flavour	Colors
1. Rose	a. Brown
2. Lemon	b. Red
3. Chocolate	c. Orange
4. Mixed fruit	d. Blue

13. Match the following:

Agents	Uses
1. Cochineal	a. Flavouring agent
2. Rose water	b. Coloring agent
3. Benzalkonium chloride	c. Antioxidant
4. Vitamin E	d. Preservatives

ANSWERS

1. 400–800 m
2. Black, colorless
3. HLB = 20 (1-saponification value/acid value)
4. Water, fat
5. Antioxidants
6. Coloring agent
7. Preservative
8. Hydrophilic lipophilic balance, Griffin
9. 3–8, 8–16
10. 1-c, 2-d, 3-b, 4-a
11. 1-b, 2-c, 3-d, 4-a
12. 1-b, 2-c, 3-a, 4-d
13. 1-b, 2-a, 3-d, 4-c.

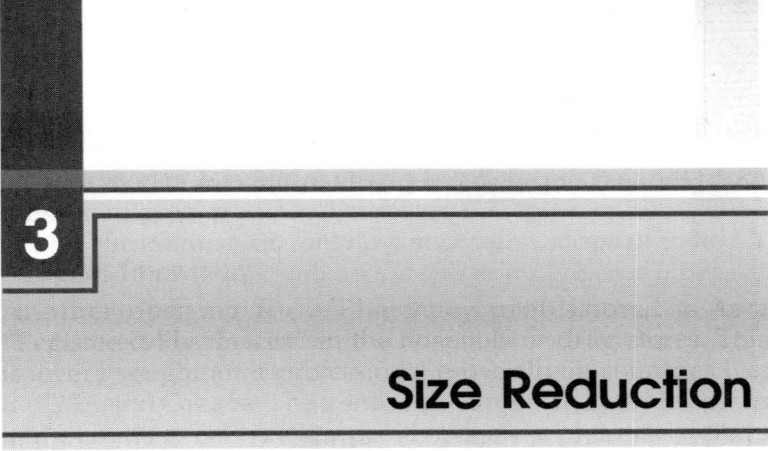

Size Reduction

Size reduction or comminution is the process of reducing the particle size of a substance to a finer state of subdivision to smaller pieces to coarse particles or to powder. When the particle size of solids is reduced by mechanical means it is known as milling. Pharmaceutical raw materials are too large to be used hence they must be reduced in size. The size reduction operation can be divided into two major categories depending on whether the material is a solid or a liquid. If the material is solid, the process is called grinding and cutting, if it is liquid, emulsification or atomization. Pharmaceutical raw materials vary in their size, shape, brittleness and toughness and the product required may vary from a coarse powder to a powder of the micron size therefore different types of size reducing machinery are used.

Importance of Particle Size Reduction

1. Size reduction increases the surface area of drugs that help in rapid dissolution.
2. Size reduction helps in extraction from animal glands such as liver and pancreas and from crude vegetable due to increase in surface area because solvent can easily penetrate into the tissues resulting in quick extraction of their active constituents.
3. The therapeutic effectiveness of certain drugs increases by reducing the particle size, e.g. the dose of griseofulvin is reduced to half.
4. The mixing of several solid ingredients is easier and more uniform if the ingredients are reduced to same particle size.

5. In the case of powdered pharmaceutical dosage forms the crystalline drugs are powdered before mixing them with other drugs in order to mix all the drugs uniformly and to avoid recognition of crystalline drugs by the patients.

6. In the manufacture of tablets API (active pharmaceutical ingredient) are mixed with excipients and made in the form of suitable size granules which are then compressed to form granules of uniform sizes.

7. The stability of emulsions is increased by decreasing the size of the oil globules.

8. Particle size plays an important role in the case of suspensions. If the size of the particles is too small, they may form a cake which may not re-disperse easily but on the other hand large size particles settle quickly but form a loose cake which may re-disperse easily on shaking.

9. It helps in the process of separation of solids from liquids by filtration or by sedimentation. The rate of filtration or sedimentation also depends upon the particle size.

10. The physical appearance of ointments, pastes and creams can be improved by reducing its particle size.

11. All the ophthalmic preparations and preparations meant for external application to the skin must be free from gritty particles to avoid irritation of the area to which they are applied.

12. The rate of absorption of a drug depends on the dosage form, route of administration and particle size. The smaller the particle size, quicker and greater will be rate of absorption.

Factors Affecting Size Reduction

1. **Hardness:** The hardness of the material affects the process of size reduction. It is easier to break soft material to a small size than hard material. An arbitrary scale of hardness has been devised known as Moh's Scale; a series of mineral substances has been given hardness numbers between 1 and 10, ranging from graphite to diamond. Up to 3 are known as soft and can be marked with the fingernail. Above 7 are hard and cannot be marked with a good pen knife blade, while those between are described as intermediate. In

general, the harder the material the more difficult it is to reduce in size.

2. **Toughness:** The crude drugs of fibrous nature or those having higher moisture content are generally tough in nature. A soft but tough material may present more problems in size reduction, than a hard but brittle substance. For example it is difficult to break rubber than a stick of blacboard chalk. Toughness is encountered in many pharmaceutical materials, particularly in fibrous drugs, and is often related to moisture content.

3. **Stickiness:** Stickiness causes a lot of difficulty in size reduction. This is due to the fact that material adheres to the grinding surfaces or sieve surface of the mill. It is difficult to powder drugs of having gummy or resinous nature, if the method used for size reduction generates heat. Complete dryness of material may help to overcome this difficulty.

4. **Material structure:** Materials which show some special structure may cause problem during size reduction, e.g. vegetable drugs which have cellular structure, generally produce long fibrous particles of its size reduction. Similarly, a mineral substance having lines of weakness, produces flake-like particles on its size reduction.

5. **Moisture content:** The presence of moisture in the material influences a number its properties such as hardness, toughness or stickiness which in its turn affects the particle size reduction. The material should be either dry or wet. It should not be damp. The material having 5% moisture in case of dry grinding and 50% moisture in wet grinding dose not create any problem.

6. **Softening temperature:** Waxy substances such as satiric acid or drugs containing oils or fats, become softened during the size reduction processes, if heat is generated. This can be avoided by cooling the mill.

7. **Purity required:** Various mills used for size reduction often cause the grinding surfaces to wear off and thus impurities come in the powder. If a high degree of purity is required, such mills must be avoided. Moreover, the mills should be thoroughly cleansed between batches of different material in order to maintain purity.

8. **Physiological effect:** Some drugs are very potent. During their particle size reduction in a mill, dust in produced which may have an effect on the operator. In such cases, the enclosed mills may be used to avoid dust.

9. **Ratio of feed size to product size:** To get a fine powder in a mill, it is required that a fairly small feed size should be used. Hence, it is necessary to carry out the size reduction process in several stages. Using different equipment, e.g. preliminary crushing following by coarse powder and then fine grinding.

10. **Bulk density:** The output of the size reduction of material in a machine, depends upon the bulk density of the substance.

Energy Requirement in Particle Size Reduction

Three laws governing energy requirements are as follows:

1. Kick's law
2. Rittinger's law
3. Bonds law

The energy required to produce a change dL in a particle of a typical size dimension is a simple power function of L as given in Equation 3.1:

$$dE/dL = KL^n \qquad \ldots (3.1)$$

Kick's Law

Kick assumed that the energy required to reduce a material in size was directly proportional to the size reduction ratio dL/L. This implies that n is equal to -1 in equation 1. Hence, Kick's law on integrating and putting the limits we get

$$E = K_K f_c \log_e (L1/L2) \qquad \ldots (3.2)$$

where,

K_K is the Kick's law constant

f_c is the crushing strength of the material

$L1$ is the feed size

$L2$ is the product size

Rittinger's Law

Rittinger, assumed that the energy required for size reduction is directly proportional, not to the change in length dimensions, but to the change in surface area. This leads to a value of -2 for n in Eqn. (3.1) as area is proportional to length squared. If we put:

$$K = K_R fc$$

and so

$$dE/dL = K_R f_c L^{-2}$$

where, K_R is called Rittinger's constant, and integrate the resulting form of Eqn. 3.1 we obtain:

$$E = K_R f_c (1/L2 - 1/L1) \qquad \qquad ... (3.3)$$

where,

$\quad\quad K_R$ is the Rittinger's constant

$\quad\quad f_c$ is the crushing strength of material

$\quad\quad L1$ is the feed size

$\quad\quad L2$ is the product size

Bond's Law

Bond has suggested an intermediate course, in which he postulates that if n is $-3/2$ in equation 1 this leads to Equation 3.4

$$E = Kb(1/(L2)^{1/2} - 1/(L1)^{1/2}) \qquad ... (3.4)$$

$$E = Ei\,(100/L2)^{1/2}\,[1 - (1/q^{1/2})] \qquad ... (3.5)$$

Bond defines the quantity Ei the work index by Equation 3.5, if L is measured in microns in above equation and so Ei is the amount of energy required to reduce unit mass of the material from an infinitely large particle size down to such a size that 80% of the product passes a 100 μm. In the above equation (3.5) q is the reduction ratio given by $q = L1/L2$. The greatest use of these equations is in making comparisons between power requirements for various degrees of reduction.

Mechanism of Size Reduction

1. **Cutting:** In this the material is cut by means of a sharp blade or blades.

2. **Compression:** In this method, the material is crushed by application of pressure.

3. **Impact:** Impact occurs when the material is more or less stationary and is hit by an object moving at high speed or when the moving particle strikes a stationary surface.

4. **Attrition:** In attrition, the material is subjected to pressure as in compression, but the surfaces are moving relative to each other, resulting in shear forces which break the particles.

5. **Attrition and impact:** In this the substances moving relative to each other hit by each other at high speed.

CRUSHER MILLS

It works on the principle of cutting. These crushers are of two types:
   a. Jaw crusher
   b. Gyratory crusher

Jaw Crusher

In a jaw crusher, the material is fed in between two heavy jaws, one fixed and the other reciprocating, so as to work the material down into a narrower and narrower space, crushing it as it goes. The **gyratory** crusher consists of a truncated conical casing, inside which a crushing head rotates eccentrically. The crushing head is shaped as an inverted cone and the material being crushed is trapped between the outer fixed, and the inner gyrating, cones, and it is again forced into a narrower and narrower space during which time it is crushed. Jaw and gyratory crusher actions are illustrated in Figs 3.1a and b. Crushing rolls consist of two horizontal heavy cylinders, mounted parallel to each other and close together. They rotate in opposite directions and the material to be crushed is trapped and nipped between them being crushed as it passes through. In some cases, the rolls are both driven at the same speed. In other cases, they may be driven at differential speeds, or only one roll is driven. A major application is in the cane sugar industry, where several stages of rolls are used to crush the cane.

ROLLER MILL

It works on the principle of attrition. Roller mills are similar to roller crushers, but they have smooth or finely fluted rolls, and

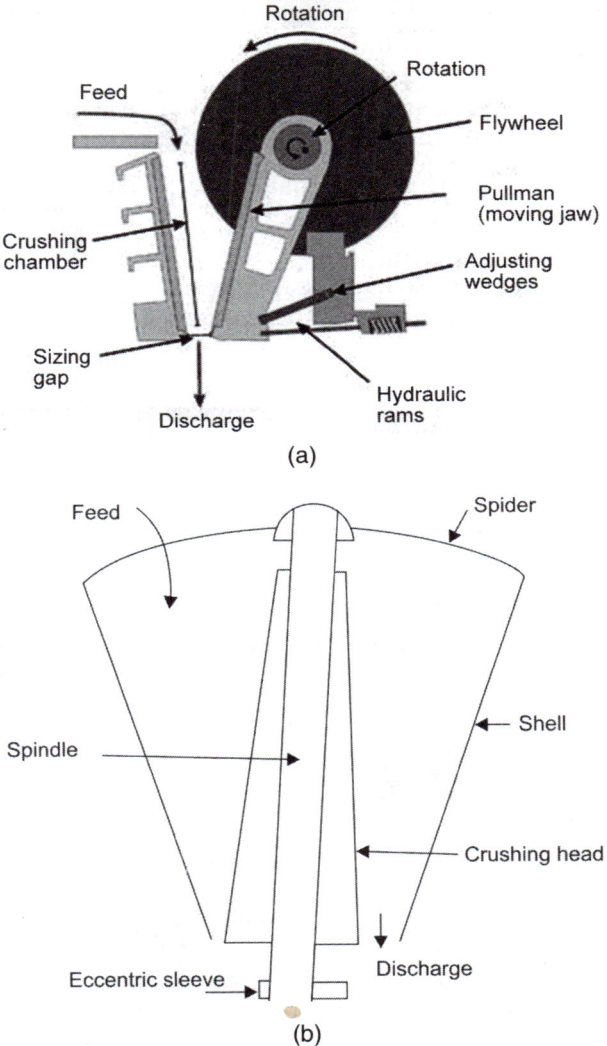

Fig. 3.1: Crushers: (a) Jaw; (b) Gyratory

rotate at differential speeds. They are used very widely to grind flour. Because of their simple geometry, the maximum size of the particle that can pass between the rolls can be regulated. If the friction coefficient between the rolls and the feed material is known, the largest particle that will be nipped between the rolls can be calculated, knowing the geometry of the particles.

The roller mills use the principles of attrition for the size reduction of solids in suspensions, pastes, or ointments. Two or three rolls, usually in metal or in porcelain, are mounted horizontally with a very small, but adjustable gap between them. The rolls rotate at different speeds, so that the material is sheared as it passes through the gap and is transferred from the slower to the faster roll, from which it is removed by means of a scraper. The method is very effective for size reducing and dispersing solids in semi-solid media.

Triple roller mill: Various types of roller mills consisting of one or more rollers are commonly used but triple roller mill is preferred. It is fitted with three rollers that are composed of a hard abrasion-resistant material. They are fitted in such a way that they come in close contact with each other and rotate at different speeds. The material that come, in-between the rollers is crushed and reduced in particle size. The reduction in particle size depends on the gap between the rollers and difference in their speeds. In Fig. 3.2, the material is allowed to pass through hopper A, in-between the rollers B and C where it is reduced

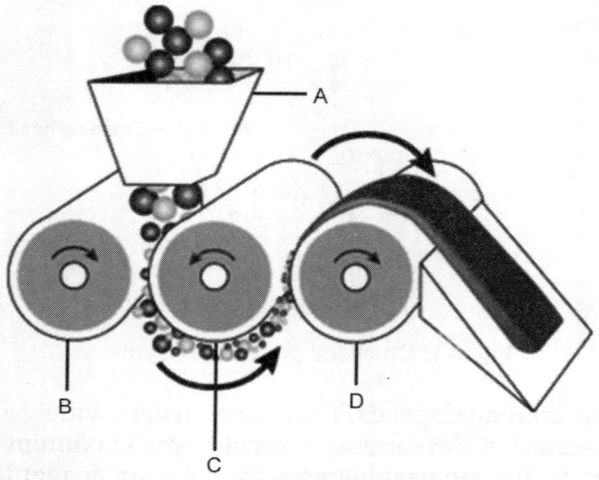

Fig. 3.2: Triple roller mill

in size. Then the material is passed between the rollers C and D where it is further reduced in size and a smooth mixture is obtained.

The gap between rollers C and D is usually less than the gap between B and C, after passing the material between rollers C and D the smoothened material is continuously removed from roller D by means of scrapper, from where it is collected in a receiver.

On large scale, mechanical ointment roller mills are used to obtain an ointment of smooth and uniform texture. The performed coarse ointments are forced to pass through moving stainless steel rollers where it is reduced in particle size and a smooth product which is uniform in composition and texture is obtained. For small scale work, small ointment mills are available.

Equipment based on the combined impact and attrition: The mechanisms of impact and attrition can be combined in two forms of mill. In the ball mill the particles receive impacts from balls or pebbles and are subjected to attrition as the balls slide over each other. In fluid energy mills the impacts and attrition occur between rapidly moving particles.

COLLOID MILL

Colloid mill works on the principle of shearing. The colloid mill is useful for milling, dispersing, homogenizing and breaking down of agglomerates in the manufacture of food pastes, emulsions, coatings, ointments, creams, pulps, grease, etc. The main function of the colloid mill is to ensure a breakdown of agglomerates or in the case of emulsions to produce droplets of fine size around 1 micron. The material to be processed is fed by gravity to the hopper or pumped so as to pass between the rotor and stator elements where it is subjected to high shearing and hydraulic forces as illustrated in Figs 3.3a and b. Material is discharged through a hopper whereby it can be recirculated for a second pass. For materials having higher solid and fiber contents conical grooved discs are preferred. Cooling and heating jacket arrangements are provided as a standard feature on both these mills.

Rotational speed of the rotor varies from 3,000 to 20,000 rpm with the spacing between the rotor and stator capable of very fine adjustment varying from 0.001 to 0.005 inch depending on

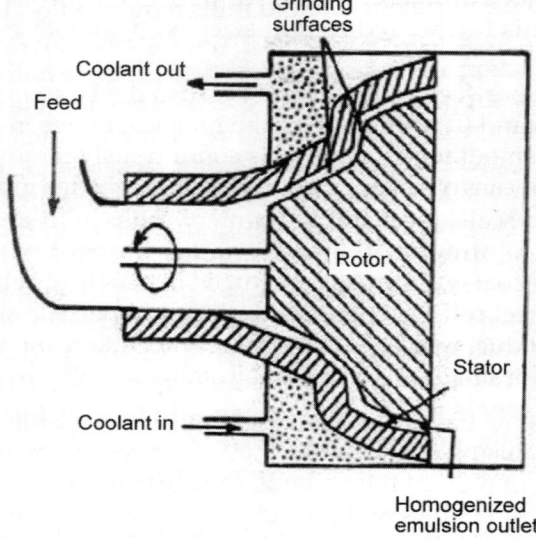

Fig. 3.3a: Premier colloid mill (conical grinding surface)

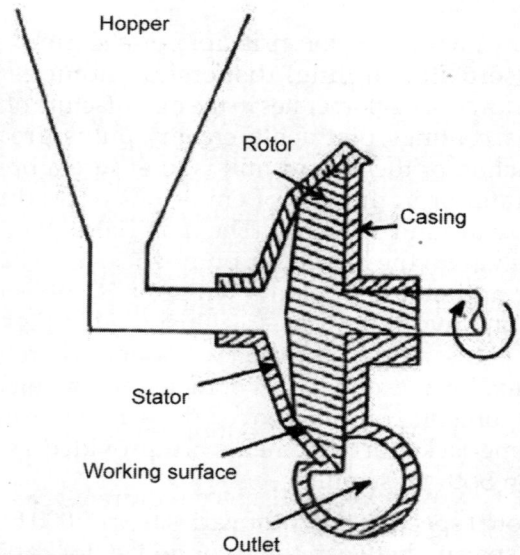

Fig. 3.3b: Colloid mill (stepped grinding surface)

the size of the equipment. Colloid mills require a flooded feed, the liquid being forced through the narrow clearance by centrifugal action and taking a spiral path. In these mills almost all the energy supplied is converted to heat and the shear forces can unduly increase the temperature of the product. Hence, most colloid mills are fitted with water jackets and it is also necessary to cool the material before and after passing through the mill. In the premier colloid mill, intense shearing action is produced between the rotor running at several thousand rpm with its working surface in close proximity to the stator. A 5-inch diameter rotor runs at 9000 rpm and has an output of 40–60 gallons depending on the viscosity of the liquid. The gap between the two surfaces is adjustable from 0.3 to 0.002 inch and the distance is measured by means of a feeler gauge. Crude mix is fed via the hopper to the center of the rotor. The material is flung outward and after homogenization across the shearing surfaces, it is discharged. If the feed is very slow, many hundreds of revolutions will take place while the contents of the gap traverse the working faces and consequently the globules will be subjected to a greater shearing action than effected at the maximum rate of feed. The materials must be supplied at such a rate that the space between the rotor and stator is kept entirely filled with liquid. Figure 3.4 shows different parts of a colloid mill.

In toothed colloid mill the grinding gap between the rotor and the stator is adjustable. Different grinding sets can be used, depending on the product. The coarse toothed set is for size reduction of solids in suspensions and coarse toothed set is for smaller particle sizes and finer dispersions. Colloid mills are used in the production of ointment, cream, gels and high viscous fluids for grinding, dispersing and homogenizing in one operation.

Advantages

- Extremely fine particle distribution through optimal shear force.
- High capacity with minimal space requirements.
- Rapid handling and easy cleaning.
- Virtually unlimited application due to highly flexible homogenization system.

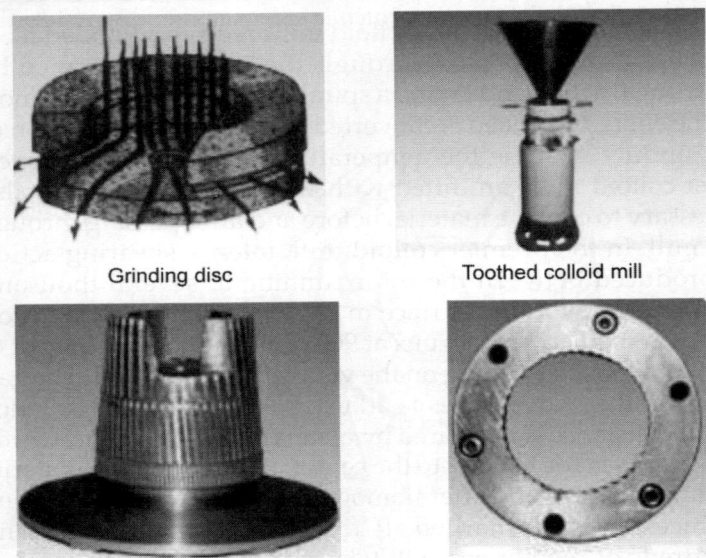

Grinding disc

Toothed colloid mill

Rotor of toothed colloid mill

Stator of toothed colloid mill

Fig. 3.4: Different parts of a colloid mill

HAMMER MILL

In the feed processing process there may be a number of ingredients that require some form of processing. These feed ingredients include coarse cereal grains, corn which require particle size reduction which will improve the performance of the ingredient and increase the nutritive value. There are a many ways to achieve this particle size reduction, here we are looking at using hammer-mills, for information on roller mills, see the related links at the bottom of this page. Both hammering and rolling can achieve the desired result of achieving adequately ground ingredients, but other factors also need to be looked at before choosing the suitable method to grind. Excessive size reduction can lead to wasted electrical energy, unnecessary wear on mechanical equipment and possible digestive problems in livestock and poultry. For more in depth information regarding what actually occurs to the ingredients during size reduction please refer to this link: Particle size reduction.

Principle *It works on the principle of impact,* i.e. the material is nearly stationary and is hitted by an object moving at a high speed (Fig. 3.5).

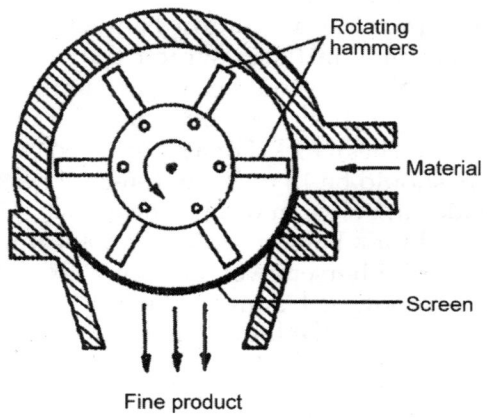

Fig. 3.5: Hammer mill

Construction and Working

The major components of these hammer mill, shown in the picture (Fig. 3.6):

1. A delivery device is used to introduce the material to be ground into the path of the hammers
2. A rotor comprised of a series of machined disks mounted on the horizontal shaft performs this task. Free-swinging hammers that are suspended from rods running parallel to the shaft and through the rotor disks. The hammers carry out the function of smashing the ingredients in order to reduce their particle size
3. A perforated screen, and
4. Gravity, or air-assisted removal of ground product

Feeder design Materials are introduced into the paths of the hammers by a variable speed vein feeder. This type of feeder can have its motor slaved by a programmable controller to the main drive motor of the hammer mill. The operational speed of the feeder is controlled to maintain optimum amperage loading of the main motor.

Hammer Design and Configuration

The design and placement of hammers is determined by operating parameters such as rotor speed, motor horsepower, and open area in the screen. Optimal hammer design and placement will provide maximum contact with the feed ingredient. Hammer mills in which the rotor speed is approximately 1,800 rpm, should be using hammers which are around 25 cm (~10 inches) long, 6.35 cm (~2.5 inches) wide, and 6.4 mm (0.25 inches) thick. For a rotor speed of about 3,600 rpm, hammers should be 15 to 20 cm (~6-8 inches long, 5 cm (~2 inches) wide, and 6.4 mm (0.25 inches) thick. The number of hammers used for a hammer mill of 1,800 rpm, should be 1 for every 2.5 to 3.5 horsepower, and for 3,600 rpm, one for every 1 to 2 horsepower. Hammers should be balanced and arranged on the rods so that they do not trail one another. The distance between hammer and screen should be 12 to 14 mm (~1/2 inch) for size reduction of cereal grains. The velocity or tip speed of the hammers is critical for proper size reduction. Tip speed is the speed of the hammer at its tip or edge furthest away from the rotor, and is calculated by multiplying the rotational speed of the drive source (shaft rpm) by the circumference of the hammer tip arc. See the following formula:

$$\text{Feet per minute} = \frac{\pi D \times \text{rpm}}{12 \text{ in/ft}}$$

π = 3.14
D = Inches diameter
rpm = Revolutions per minute

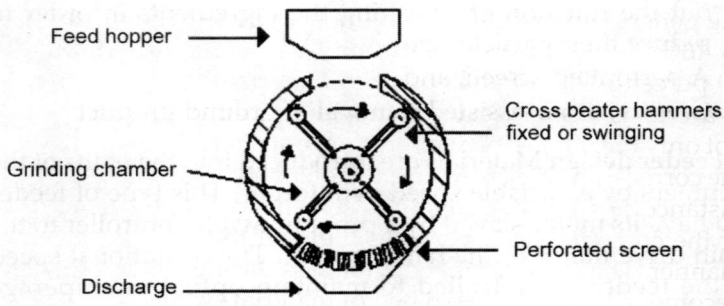

Fig. 3.6: Major components of hammer mill

A common range of tip speeds seen in hammer mills is commonly in the range between 5,000 and 7,000 m/min (~16,000 and 23,000 feet per minute). When the tip speeds exceed 23,000 feet per minute, careful consideration must be given to the design of the hammer mill, the materials used in its construction, and the fabrication of all the components. Simply changing the rotational speed of the drive source is not a recommended method of increasing hammer speed in excess of 23,000 feet per minute. Impact is the primary force used in a hammer mill. Anything which increases the chance of a collision between a hammer and a target; increases the magnitude of the collision; or improves material take-away provides an advantage in particle size reduction. The magnitude of the collisions can be escalated by increasing the speed of the hammers.

Screen Design

The amount of open area in a hammer mill screen determines the particle size and grinding efficiency. The screen must be designed to maintain its integrity and provide the greatest amount of open area. Screen openings (holes) that are aligned in a 60-degree staggered pattern optimize open area while maintaining screen strength. This method will result in a 40 percent open area using 3.2 mm (1/8 inch) holes aligned on 4.8 mm (3/16 inch) centers.

Feed producers need to pay particular attention to the ratio of open screen area to horsepower. Recommended ratio for grains would be 55 cm^2 (~8–9 inches square) per horsepower (Bliss, 1990). Not enough open area per horsepower results in the generation of heat. When the heat generated exceeds 44C to 46C (120–125F), capacity may be decreased as much as 50 percent. The removal of sized material from a hammermill is a critical design feature. Proper output of material affects not only the efficiency of operation, but also particle size. When the correct ratio of screen area to horsepower is used and proper distance between hammers and screen face is maintained, most of the correctly sized particles will exit the screen in a timely manner. The particles that do not pass through the screen holes become part of a fluidized bed of material swept along the face of the screen by the high-speed rotation of the hammers. As these particles rub against the screen and each other their size is continually reduced by attrition. This excessive size reduction is counterproductive. Energy is wasted in the production of heat, throughput is restricted, and particles become too small.

Most newer hammer mills are equipped with an air-assist system that draws air into the hammer mill with the product to be ground. Systems are designed to provide reduced pressure on the exit side of the screen to disrupt the fluidized bed of material on the face of the screen, thus allowing particles to exit through screen holes. Some full circle hammer mills are designed so the screen is in two pieces. It is possible to use a larger hole size on the upward arc of the hammers to further reduce the amount of material on the face of the screen.

Hammers are used inside the hammer mill to impact smash ingredients up into smaller particles, making it more suitable for uniform mixing and usage in feed. Hammers are available in a huge range of configurations, shapes, facings and materials. Hammers are available as single holed or with two holes, with two holes allowing the hammers to be used twice as the wear is done to one end of the hammer, the hammer can be rotated and used a second time. The hole fits onto a rod inside the hammer mill and swings to hit the material.

Dimensions of a hammer which play role in size reduction are:

  A: Thickness
  B: Width
  C: Diameter to fit rod size
  D: Swing length
  E: Total length

Hammer mills screens are used inside a hammer mill to seperate particle sizes (Fig. 3.7). Particle of small enough diameter that has been successfully grinded by the hammer mill passes through the screen and leaves the hammer mill with the help of the pneumatic system.

Size reduction: The initial reduction of cereal grains begins by disrupting the outer protective layer of the seed (hull), exposing the interior (Fig. 3.8). Continued size reduction increases both the number of particles and the amount of surface area per unit of volume. It is this increased surface area

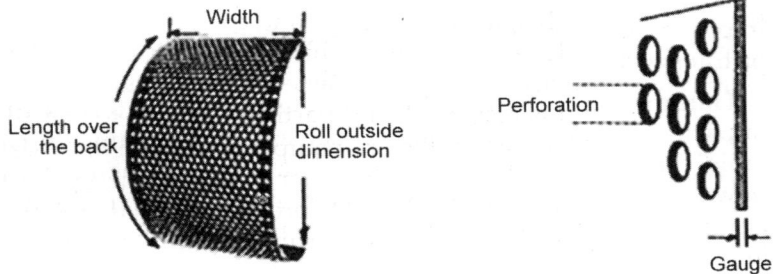

Fig. 3.7: Hammer mill screen

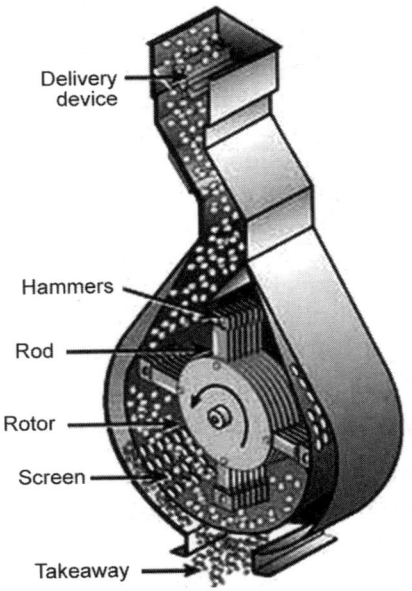

Fig. 3.8: Interior of hammer mill

that is of primary importance. A greater portion of the grain's interior is exposed to digestive enzymes, allowing increased access to nutritional components such as starch and protein. The enhanced breakdown of these nutritional components improves absorption in the digestive tract. The overall effect is increased animal performance. Size reduction is also used to modify the physical characteristics of ingredients resulting in improved mixing, pelleting, and, in some instances, handling or transport.

Hammer mills reduce the particle size of materials by impacting a slow moving target, such as a cereal grain, with a rapidly moving hammer. The target has a little or no momentum (low kinetic energy), whereas the hammer tip is traveling at a minimum of 4,880 m/min (~16,000 feet per min) and perhaps in excess of 7,015 m/min (~23,000 feet per min) (high kinetic energy). The transfer of energy that results from this collision fractures the grain into many pieces. Sizing is a function of hammer-tip speed; hammer design and placement; screen design and hole size; and whether or not air assistance is utilized.

Because impact is the primary force used in a hammer mill to reduce the size of the particles, anything that; increases the chance of a collision between a hammer and a target, increases the magnitude of the collision, or improves material takeaway, would be advantageous to particle size reduction. The magnitude of the collisions can be escalated by increasing the speed of the hammers. Particles produced using a hammer mill will generally be spherical in shape with a surface that appears polished. The distribution of particle sizes will vary widely around the geometric mean such that there will be some large-sized and many small-sized particles.

Advantages of Hammer Mill

- Are able to produce a wide range of particle sizes
- Work with any friable material and fiber
- Ease of use
- Lower initial investment when compared with a roller mill
- Minimal maintenance needed
- Particles produced using a hammermill will generally be spherical, with a surface that appears polished.

Disadvantages of Hammer Mill

- Less energy efficient when compared to a roller mill
- May generate heat (source of energy loss)

- Produce greater particle size variability (less uniform)
- Hammer mills are noisy and can generate dust pollution

Uses: The hammer mill is used for producing intermediate grades of powder from almost all type of substances except sticky materials that choke the screen.

BALL MILL

Principle: It works on the principle of impact and attrition.

Construction: It consists of hollow cylinder mounted on a metallic frame in such a way that it can rotate horizontally on its axis. The cylinder contain balls that occupy 30–50% of the mill volume. The weight of the balls is kept constant. The ball size depends on the size of the feed and the diameter of the mill. The cylinder and balls are made of metal and are usually lined with chrome. In pharmaceutical industry, sometimes the cylinder of ball mill is lined with rubber or porcelain. The balls used in these mills are also made of rubber or porcelain (Fig. 3.9).

Working: The drug to be ground is put into the cylinder of the mill and is roated. The speed of rotation is very important.

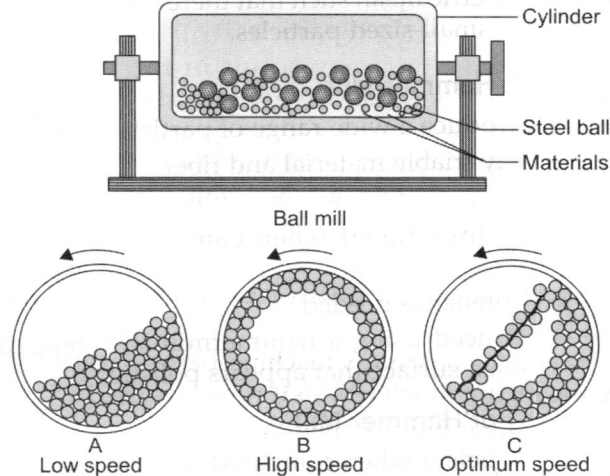

Ball mill

A — Low speed
B — High speed
C — Optimum speed

Fig. 3.9: Ball mill and its working

At a low speed, the mass of balls with will slide or roll over each other and only a negligible amount of size reduction will occur. At a high speed, the balls will be thrown out to the balls by centrifugal force and no grinding will occur. But at about 2/3rd of the speed, the centrifugal force just occurs with result that the balls are carried almost to the top of the mill and then fall in. By this way the maximum size reduction is effected by the impact of particles between the balls and by attrition between the balls. After a suitable time, the material is taken out and passed through a sieve to get powder of the required size.

Advantages of Ball Mill

1. It can produce very fine powders.
2. It can be used for continuous operation, if sieve or classifier is attached to the mill.
3. It is capable of grinding a large variety of materials of different characters and of different degree of hardness.
4. It is suitable for both wet and dry grinding processes.
5. It can be used to grind toxic materials as it can be used in a completely enclosed form.

Disadvantages of Ball Mill

1. Wear occurs, principally from the balls, but partially from the casing and this may result in the product being contaminated, with abrasive materials this may exceed 0.1 percent, but even ordinary substances may be contaminated with 0.03 percent metal after grinding.
2. In some cases, this may not be significant, but in others it may be of a great importance.
3. Soft or sticky materials may cause problems by caking on the sides of the mill or by holding the balls in aggregates.
4. The ball mill is very noisy machine, particularly if the casing is of metal, but much less so if rubber is used.
5. Relatively long time of operation.

Uses: Ball mills are applicable to a wide variety of materials, large ones being used for grinding ores prior to manufacture of pharmaceutical chemicals and small versions for the final grinding of drugs or for grinding suspensions.

FLUID ENERGY MILL

Principle: *It works on the principle of impact and attrition.* The fluid energy mill employs no moving parts—size reduction results from attrition between rapidly moving particles of the material being ground. The energy to achieve these high particle velocities is supplied by a compressed fluid, normally air, gas or steam, which enters the grinding chamber at high speeds through purpose designed nozzles in the periphery.

Features of the Fluid Energy Mill

1. Production of fine particles in the lower micron range: Normally particle with an average size of less than 5 microns are possible.

2. Flexibility: The operation of the mill may be simply and rapidly altered to suit different products and also obtain varying grades of material from coarse to fine particle sizes.

3. Ease of cleaning and sterilizing: The mill is designed for efficient and easy cleaning and so is especially suitable for operating on various substances in quick succession.

4. Narrow particle size spectrum: The range of particle size in the product is very much smaller than with any other type of mill today.

5. Dustless operation.

6. Temperature control: Absence of moving parts and the cooling effect due to the expansion of compressed fluids leaving the jets, enables heat sensitive products to be easily processed.

7. Uniformity of products: Controlled operating conditions with intense classifying action produces a high-degree of uniformity in the product.

8. Single cycle operation: The production of lower micron particle sizes is achieved with only one pass through the mill.

9. Variation of particle size: Product particle size can be controlled and varied. Products and processes are improved and standards of purity increased.

Construction and Working

It consist of a loop of pipe, which has diameter of 20 to 200 mm, depending on the overall height of the loop, which may be up to about 2 m. There is an inlet for the feed and a series of nozzles for the inlet of air or an inert gas. It also has an outlet with a classifier which allows the air to escape but prevents the particles to pass until they become sufficiently fine.

The fluid energy mill comprises essentially of a flat horizontal cylindrical chamber, equipped with tangentially arranged jet nozzles in the inner wall (Fig. 3.10). The energy for milling is provided with a compressed fluid such as compressed air, or in the case where materials being milled provide a risk of a dust explosion, gaseous nitrogen. The compressed fluid issues through the nozzles forming a very high velocity tangential circle within the grinding chamber. The feed material is injected into that same tangential circle via a venturi feeder, where it is rapidly accelerated, causing it to impact against itself, thus fracturing the particles to the low micron range. Larger particles

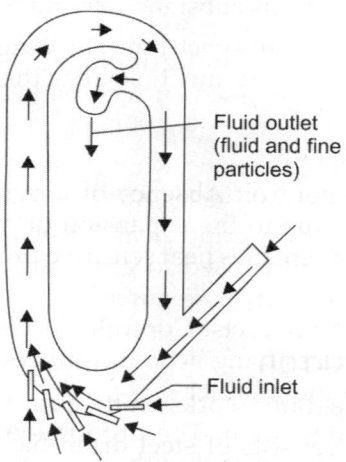

Fig. 3.10: Fluid energy mill

are held by centrifugal force towards the outer periphery of the chamber, while the smaller particles travel, in a spiral movement toward the center, from where they exit either into a cyclone below for bottom discharge, or through the top of the mill into a reverse pulse product/filter system.

Advantages of Fluid Energy Mill

- The mill is used to grind the material to fine powder.
- The particle size of powder can be controlled due to the use of a classifier.
- There is no wear of the mill and hence there is no contamination of the product.
- It is useful for grinding heat sensitive substance such as sulphonamides, vitamins and antibiotics.

Uses

Many materials have been successfully processed in the fluid energy mills including food products, pharmaceuticals, chemicals, antibiotics, plastics, pigments, dyes, fungicides, insecticides, powdered metals, cosmetics, organic and inorganic materials, non-metallic minerals and ores.

The design of the fluid energy mill enables other processes and functions to be carried out such as:

1. Intimate mixing or coating one material with another while simultaneously grinding and classifying.
2. Simultaneous drying and grinding of moist materials by using heated compressed air or superheated steam.
3. Reduction of materials suspended in liquids.
4. Certain chemical reactions, which have a direct relationship with micron, sized particles, such as oxidation.
5. The mill is used to grind heat sensitive material to fine powder. The mill is used to grind those drugs in which high degree of purity is required.

THE DISINTEGRATOR

Principle: Disintegrator works on the principle of impact.

Construction: It consists of steel drum having a shaft in the center. The shaft contain a disc, on which four to five beater are fixed. The shaft rotates with a speed of 5000–7000 rev/min the side and upper inner surface of the drum is rough and undulating. The lower part of the drum has a detached screen or sieve having a definite pore size (Fig. 3.11).

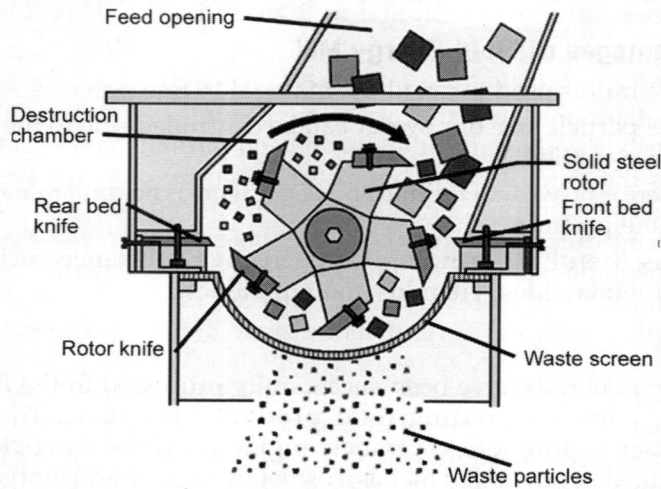

Fig. 3.11: The disintegrator

Working: The material to be reduced in size is fed from the feed opening. It comes in contact with the moving solid steel rotor (beater).

The beater is mainly responsible for grinding but is helped by the wave of inner surface and roughness of drum. As material is fed into the unit it falls down a chute into a destruction chamber which contains a rotor with 4–5 knives mounted to it. The rotating knives pass by 2 stationary bed knives (rear bed knife and front bed knife) and cut the waste smaller and smaller with each pass. The material is broken into small particles by impact and cutting of the beaters. The fine particles produced passes through the screen located at the bottom while the bigger particles remain inside the destruction chamber which further get reduced by the beaters.

Use: The mill is used to powder all type of drugs including very hard drugs. The drug should be dried properly before feeding into disintegrator to get fine powder. To avoid the jamming of the beaters of the disintegrator, use moderately small pieces of drug particles. This method of grinding is very efficient for a wide range of dry materials and in some cases, also for wet materials.

Factors Influencing Choice of Size Reduction Machinery

1. **Nature of the raw material:** Drugs must be thoroughly dried before they are subjected to size reduction. Drugs like belladonna, gentian, liquorice and squill are returned to the drying rooms after they have been partially comminuted, as they rapidly absorb moisture from the atmosphere and as the moisture may not be removed from all parts of the drug during the initial drying stage. In the case of water insoluble substances, wet grinding of the material can be done. For the preparation of aqueous dispersions of drugs this method is very effective since deflocculating agents may be included to prevent agglomeration of the particles. Substances that are hygroscopic or volatile or very poisonous or that need-prolonged trituration are more easily prepared in closed porcelain ball mills. Fibrous material seed tearing apart of the fibers and this can be achieved in high-speed impact mills. Substances of a resinous or oily nature shall not be subjected to heavy pressures or much heat as a pasty mass may result. Hence, a ball mill will not be suitable and they are better grounded in a micronizer or a hammer mill. The replacement of air by an inert gas is necessary when grinding readily oxidizable materials and ball mills and high-speed impact mills are generally used in this way.

2. **Nature of the product:** A powdered drug produced in a ball mill differs from the product in a micronizer or a disintegrator even though both powders may be screened to the same fineness. Differences exist in the shape of the particles, their toughness and their internal pore structure. Powder obtained from grinding mills like ball mill is more compact and less porous than that obtained in high speed impact mills like a disintegrator. For the grinding of a sterile material under aseptic conditions, a mill is required that can be easily sterilized and sealed to prevent contamination during the grinding operation. A batch operation porcelain

ball mill is most suitable for this purpose. When iron and copper contamination of pharmaceutical products is to be avoided stainless steel or ceramic material may be used for the surfaces of a mill coming into contact with the drug.

3. **Degree of comminution required:** The degree of comminution of materials varies according to the purpose for which they are required. For the preparation of galenicals, the size of the vegetable drug powder employed for extraction varies from coarse to fine powder. Tincture preparation requires bruised to moderately coarse powders. For percolation, drug powders should not contain a large proportions of fines to avoid uneven extraction. Coarse to moderately coarse powder, with a minimum of fine powder, are all most easily obtained by using high speed mills of the impact type. Materials such as cascara, liquorice, belladonna leaf and root and ginger are all easily broken down in such mills. The grindability of different grades of a vegetable drug usually varies and during comminution the softer portions get size reduced first. Therefore, it is sometimes useful to screen out the powdered drug and return the coarser material to the mill for further size reduction. This prevents continued milling of the softer portions resulting in formation of too much fines. The same principle is also applicable to crystalline drugs although they are of uniform composition. The rate of absorption of sparingly soluble drugs, either through the gastrointestinal tract or when administered parenterally, depends on particle size. Penicillin in a medium of aluminium monostearte and arachis oil appears to be most effective when 90% of the particles are smaller than 5 micrometers. The relatively insoluble sulphonamides attain their maximum antibacterial activity at crystal sizes of about 1 micrometer or below. For insufflations the drug should be smaller than about 5 micrometers.

Pharmaceutical Applications of Size Reduction

- Size reduction increases the surface area per unit weight also known as the specific surface area. This increased specific surface affects the therapeutic efficiency of medicinal compounds that possess a low solubility in body fluids by increasing the area of contact between the solids and the

Table 3.1: Characteristics of various type of mills and their action

Sr. No.	Name of mill	Principle	Mess size	Uses	Not used for
1	Cutter mill	Cutting	20–80	Fibrous and crude drug	Friable drug
2	Roller mill	Compression	20–200	Soft drugs	Hard drugs
3	Hammer mill	Impact	4–325 a	Almost ll drugs	Soft and sticky drugs
4	Disintegrator	Impact	20–80	Brittle and hard drugs	Soft drugs
5	Ball mill and impact	Attrition	20–200	Brittle and hard drugs	Soft and malleable drugs
6	Fluid energy mill	Attrition and impact	1–30 micron	Hard and friable drugs	Soft and sticky substance

dissolving fluid. Thus, a given weight of finely powdered medicinal compound dissolves in a shorter time than does the same weight of a coarse powder. For example, the control of fineness of griseofulvin led to an oral dosage regimen half that of the originally marketed product.

- Particle size control influences the duration of adequate serum concentration, rheology, and product syringeability of a suspension of penicillin G procaine for intramuscular injection.
- The rectal absorption of aspirin from a theobroma oil suppository is related to particle size.
- There is an increase in antiseptic action for calomel ointment when the particle size of calomel is reduced.
- The size of particles used in inhalation aerosols determines the position and retention of the particles in the bronchopulmonary system.
- Size may affect texture, taste and rheology of oral suspensions in addition to absorption.
- The time required for dissolution of solid chemicals in the preparation of solutions is shortened by the use of smaller particles.

PRACTICE QUESTIONS

Q. 1. Enumerate the various factors which affect the size reduction of drugs.

Q. 2. Give the advantage of ball mill.

Q. 3. Write the advantage of fluid energy mill.

Q. 4. Describe the various laws governing size reduction.

Q. 5. What are the various mechanism of size reduction?

Q. 6. Explain the principle, construction and working of ball Mill.

Q. 7. Describe the principle, construction and working of hammer mill. What are its advantages and disadvantages?

Q. 8. How does stickiness and moisture affects the process of size reduction?

Q. 9. Write the significance of size reduction in pharmacy.

Q. 10. Explain the construction and working of disintegrator with the help of a neat and labeled diagram.

Q. 11. Compare and contrast working of ball mill and hammer mill.

Q. 12. Describe the construction and working of a fluid energy mill with the help of neat diagram.

OBJECTIVE TYPE QUESTIONS

1. Cutter mill works on the principle of ....
....

2. Hammer mill works on the principle of ....
....

3. Ball mill works on the principle of ....

4. Fluid energy mill works on the principle of ....

5. The efficiency of ball mill is maximum at .... of its speed

6. Particle size reduction .... the surface area of solid substance

7. Match the following:

Type of mill	Mess size
1. Ball mill	a. 20–80
2. Hammer mill	b. 20–200
3. Disintegrator	c. 1–30 μ
4. Fluid energy mill	d. 4–325

ANSWERS

1. Cutting

2. Impact

3. Attrition and impact

4. Attrition and impact

5. 2/3

6. Increases

7. 1-b, 2-d, 3-a, 4-c

4

Size Separation

The control of particles size and size range is of a great importance in pharmaceutical industry. Though various types of machines are used for size reduction, it is not necessary that they will produce the desired size particles and of uniform size. Any solid material, after size reduction, never gives particles of the same size but contains particles of somewhat varying sizes. To control the particle size distribution, the size-reduced material must be sifted to sifting to get fractions of narrow size ranges. The desired fractions are finally mixed, if necessary, in such a way to get a powder having the needed average particle size. Thus, one can say that size separation is usually an integral part of size reduction in industrial pharmacy. After the drug has been subjected to size reduction, the powered drug is separated according to its particle size. The various methods used for size separation are:

1. Sieving
2. Cyclone separator
3. Air separator
4. Elutriation

SIEVING

In this method, the fine powder is separated from the coarse powder by using sieve of desired number. The degree of fineness of powder is known with the help of sieve through which the powder material is passed. Sieves are numbered in order to distinguish them from each other (Fig. 4.1).

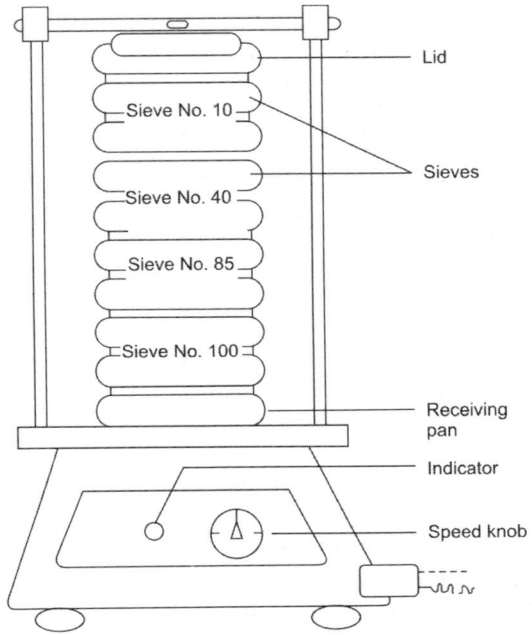

Fig. 4.1: Multiple sieving machine

Size separation of powder is done by passing the powdered material through a set of sieve. The larger size is at the top and the smallest one at the bottom. The bottom sieve is attached to the receiving pan. The material is placed in the upper most sieve.

The working of mechanical sieving devices are based on any of the following method:

1. Agitation
2. Brushing
3. Centrifugal

1. **Agitation method:** Sieves may be agitated in a number of different ways, such as:

 a. *Oscillation:* The sieves are mounted in a frame that oscillates back and forth.

 b. *Vibration:* The sieves are vibrated at high speed by means of an electric device. The rapid vibration is imparted to the particles on the sieves which help to pass. The powdered material through it.

c. *Gyration:* In this method, a system is made so that sieve is on rubber mounting and connected to an eccentric fly wheel. This give a rotary movement of small amplitude to sieve, which in turns, give spinning motion to the particle that help to pass them through the sieve.

Agitation method are not continuous method but can be made so by inclination of the sieve and the provision of separate outlets for under sieve and over sieve particle.

2. **Brushing method:** In this method, a brush is used to move the particle on the surface of the sieve and to keep the meshes clear. The brush is rotated in the middle in the case of circular sieve but spiral brush is rotated on the longitudinal axis in case of a horizontal cylindrical sieve.

3. **Centrifugal method:** In this method, a high speed rotor is fixed inside the vertical cylindrical sieve, so that on the rotator of rotor, the particles are thrown outward by centrifugal force. The current of air which is produced due to high speed of rotor helps in sieving the powder.

On shaking the powdered material in a mechanical or electromagnetic device using any of the above methods, the weight of power retained on each sieve is determined. The percentage of each fraction is then calculated.

Materials Used for Sieves

The only official specification for materials for the construction of sieves is that the wire should be of uniform, circular cross-section. In addition, however, the material should have suitable strength to avoid distortion and be resistant to corrosion by any substances that may be shifted.

1. Metals

a. **Iron:** Iron wire has the advantage because its cheap, but it has a disadvantage that rusting occurs very readily and iron contamination of products is usually undesirable.

Coated iron: Iron wire may be coated as a protection from corrosion by galvanizing or tinning, but there is a tendency for the diameter to become variable. Some sieves are coated after manufacture, which increases the protection against corrosion and increases the strength also, but is likely to lead to some variation in the mesh size. Like all coatings, it remains effective, if it is not damaged.

b. **Copper:** Copper wire is readily available and is used commonly. Copper has the advantage that it avoids the risk of iron contamination, but it is a soft metal and the meshes can be distorted easily.

Copper alloys: A number of alloys of copper, for example brass and phosphorus-bronze, resemble copper in possessing good resistance to corrosion by most materials but strength is very much greater so that there is less risk of the meshes being distorted in use.

c. **Stainless steel:** Stainless steel is the most expensive of the metals from which sieves are made, stainless steel is the most satisfactory, having good resistance to corrosion by all materials that are likely to be sieved, as well as adequate strength. Sieves with stainless steel meshes are recommended for pharmaceutical purposes for the above reasons.

2. **Non-metals:** Sieves with meshes from non-metals are used when it is important that all risk of metallic contamination be avoided. Non-metals are used also in sieves with fine meshes, since many non-metal fibers are stronger than a metal wire of comparable thickness.

Materials of natural origin, for example hair and silk, were used originally, but synthetic fibers have proved to be more satisfactory. Man-made fibers, such as nylon and terylene, are excellent, having considerable strength and resistance to corrosion. In addition, these materials can be extruded in all diameters, enabling a wide variety of sieves to be made.

Advantages of Sieving

- It is a quick and reliable method of size analysis, equally suited to accurate scientific research work or routine analysis under industrial conditions.
- Tests can be performed at almost any location.

- No complicated apparatus is demanded. A nest of sieves and a simple laboratory balance is sufficient.
- No specialized knowledge or skill is needed; care and diligence are the main requirements.
- When the size distribution of a sample has been determined by test sieving, the material becomes separated into several fractions. This is another important attribute. These fractions are not contaminated, nor have their chemical or physical properties been altered.
- The equipment used for sieving is not expensive.

Official Standards for Powders

The Indian Pharmacopoeia has laid down the standards for powders for pharmaceutical purposes. According to IP, the degree of coarseness or fineness of powder is expressed with reference to the nominal mesh aperture size of the sieve through which powder is able to pass.

The IP specifies five grades of powder which are as under:

1. **Coarse powder:** When all the particles of powder pass through a sieve with nominal mesh aperture of 1.70 mm (No. 10 sieve) and not more than 40.0% through a sieve with nominal mesh aperture of 355 mm (No. 44 sieve) is called coarse powder.

2. **Moderately coarse powder:** When all the particles of powder pass through a sieve with nominal mesh aperture of 710 mm (No. 22 sieve) and not more than 40.0% through a sieve with nominal mesh aperture of 250 mm (No. 60 sieve) is called moderately coarse powder.

3. **Moderately fine powder:** When all the particles of powder pass through a sieve with nominal mesh aperture of 355 mm (No. 44 sieve) and not more than 40.0% through a sieve with nominal mesh aperture of 180 mm (No. 85 sieve), is called moderately fine powder.

4. **Fine powder:** When all the particles of powder pass through a sieve with a normal mesh aperture of 180 mm (No. 85 sieve), it is called fine powder.

5. **Very fine powder:** When all the particles of powder pass through a sieve with a nominal mesh aperture of 125 mm (No. 120 sieve), it is said to be very fine powder.

The relevant grades of powder and sieve numbers along with a nominal mesh aperture are shown in Table 4.1.

Table 4.1: Type of powder and its various characteristics

S. No.	Type of powder	Sieve number (all particles must pass)	Nominal mesh aperture size	Sieve number (40% of particles must pass)	Mesh aperture size
1.	Coarse powder	10	1.7 mm	44	355 mm
2.	Moderately coarse powder	22	710 mm	60	250 mm
3.	Moderately fine powder	44	355 mm	85	180 mm
4.	Fine powder	85	180 mm	–	–
5.	Very fine powder	120	125 mm	–	–

SIEVES

Sieves for pharmacopoeia testing are constructed from wire cloth with square meshes, woven from wires of brass, bronze, stainless steel or any other suitable material. The wires should be of uniform circular cross-section and should not be coated or plated. There should not be any reaction between the material of the sieve and the substance which is being sifted from it.

Standards for sieves: Sieves used for pharmacopoeia testing must specify the following:

1. **Number of sieve:** Sieve number indicates the number of meshes in a length of 2.54 cm. In each transverse direction parallel to the wires.

2. **Nominal size of aperture:** Nominal size of aperture indicates the distance between the wires. It represents the length of the side of the square aperture. The IP has given

the nominal mesh aperture size for majority of sieves in mm.

3. **Nominal diameter of the wire:** Wire mesh sieves are made from the wire having the specified diameter in order to give a suitable aperture size and sufficient strength to avoid deformation of the sieve.

4. **Approximate percentage sieving area:** This standard expresses the area of the meshes as a percentage of the total area of the sieve. It depends on the size of the wire used for any particular sieve number. Generally the sieving area is kept within the range of 35 to 40% in order to give suitable strength to the sieve.

5. **Tolerance average aperture size:** Some variation in the aperture size is unavoidable and when this variation is expressed as a percentage, it is known as the 'aperture tolerance average'. In fact, it is a limit given by pharmacopoeia within which a particular dimension or average aperture size can be allowed to very and still be acceptable for the purpose for which it is used. Fine meshes cannot be woven with the same accuracy as coarse meshes. Hence, the aperture tolerance average is smaller for coarse sieves than the fine sieves. According to IP a sieve must confirm to the following specifications as given in Table 4.2.

Factors Affecting the Efficiency of A Sieving System

Rate of feeding: If feed rate is too high, there is insufficient residence time. The screen becomes overloaded, and some "fines" leave with the oversize.

Particle size: Large particles can impede the path of smaller ones, and a preliminary separation may be required if a high proportion of larger particles are present.

Moisture: Moisture can cause adhesion of small particles to larger ones, so some undersize leave with the oversize.

Worn or damaged screens: Oversize may fall through damaged areas.

Blinding (clogging) of screens: Particularly likely when the size of particles is very close to the screen aperture. Result can be undersize leaving with oversize.

Table 4.2: Sieve number there mesh aperture and there tolerance average aperture size

S. No.	Approximate sieve number	Approximate percentage sieving area	Nominal mesh aperture size (mm)	Tolerance average aperture size ($\pm$ mm)
1	4	55	4.0	0.13
2	6	1	2.8	0.09
3	8	48	2.0	0.07
4	10	46	1.7	0.06
5	˙12	44	1.4	0.05
6	16	41	1.0	0.03
7	–	–	mm	$\pm$ mm
8	22	37	710	25
9	25	36	600	21
10	30	38	500	18
11	36	36	425	15
12	44	38	355	13
13	60	37	250	13 (9.9)
14	85	35	180	11 (7.6)
15	100	36	150	9.4 (6.6)
16	120	34	125	8.1 (5.8)
17	150	36	106	7.4 (5.2)
18	170	35	90	6.6 (4.6)
19	200	36	75	6.1 (4.1)
20	240	34	63	5.3 (3.7)
21	300	35	53	4.8 (3.4)
22	350	34	45	4.8 (3.1)

Electrostatic charge: When screening dry powders, surfaces can become charged, resulting in small particles clumping together and leaving with the oversize. Grounding of screens may be necessary.

Stokes' Law

Stokes' law is a formula for determining the rate of sedimentation. It states that a particle moving through viscous liquid attains a constant velocity or sedimentation rate. The rate can be very slow for particles whose density is close to that of the liquid, for particles whose diameter is small, or where the viscosity is high. Replacing gravitational acceleration with the acceleration generated by a rotating centrifuge results in faster sedimentation. Centrifugal acceleration can be thousands of times greater than that of gravity, so the centrifugal sedimentation rate is thousands of times greater.

The following is the equation for Stokes' law of sedimentation:

$$V_g = d^2 \, (P_p - P_1)/18\mu \times G$$

where,

V_g = Sedimentation velocity

d = Particle diameter

P_p = Particle density

P_1 = Liquid density

G = Gravitational acceleration

μ = Viscosity of liquid

Sedimentation uses gravitational forces to separate particulate material from fluid streams. The particles are usually solid, but they can be small liquid droplets, and the fluid can be either a liquid or a gas. Sedimentation is very often used in the food industry for separating dirt and debris from incoming raw material, crystals from their mother liquor and dust or product particles from air streams.

SIZE SEPARATION BY SETTLING

When particles are too small to be screened effectively or when large quantities of material are to be handled, methods involving differences in the rates of settling of particles of different sizes and of different materials are used. If two particles of different settling rates in water are placed in an upward flowing stream and if the velocity of water is adjusted so that it lies between the settling rates of the two particles, the slowing settling particles will move downward against the water stream and a separation is thereby obtained as illustrated in Fig. 4.2.

Consider there are two particles having different settling rates admitted horizontally into a small tank containing water,

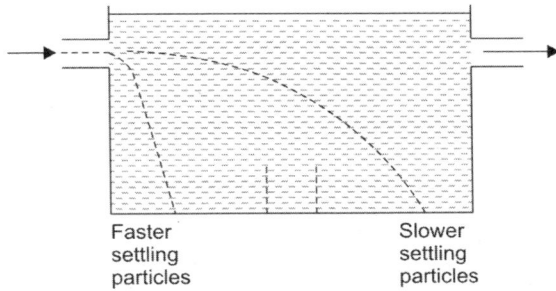

Faster
settling
particles

Slower
settling
particles

Fig. 4.2: Simple hydraulic separation

both particles start to settle. The faster settling particle reaches the bottom of the tank before the slower moving particle. The settling rates of a particle depends both on their size and their shapes. Since the water velocities in any one cross-section of the above classifying devices are not uniform, with particles of uniform density but varying in size and shape, the methods do not give fractions having all the particles in a relatively small size range but rather fractions having a mixture of sizes with the average size smaller in one fraction and larger in the other. Hence, these procedures are called *classification methods* rather than size separation methods. The settling rate of a particle also depends on its density. If the material to be classified is a mixture of materials of different densities and sizes, the coarser fraction will be richer in the heavier component and the finer fractions will be richer in the lighter component. Classification equipment may involve simple settling as above or the settling may be aided by mechanical devices. The system may operate only on the water entering with the material or a stream of additional water may be supplied. This additional water is called hydraulic water, if the apparatus is to settle out all the solids introduced and give a clear overflow, the process is called sedimentation.

SEDIMENTATION METHODS

Sedimentation methods are based on the measurement of the rate at which particles of the powder settle out from a liquid in which they have been dispersed. The pipet method (Andreason) as shown in Fig. 4.3, is the simplest means of incremental

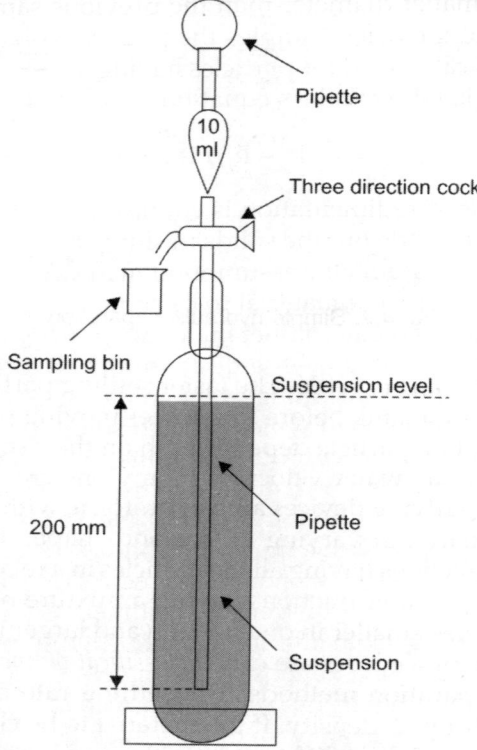

Fig. 4.3: Andreason pipette

particle size analysis. The Andreason apparatus consists of a tall vessel called sedimentation vessel having capacity of 500 ml. The vessel is fitted with groundglass joint through which a 10-ml pipette fitted with two-way stopcock for draining sample is passed. A 1% suspension of the powder is prepared in a suitable liquid medium which is then placed in the sedimentation vessel. As measured by the pipette 10 ml samples are withdrawn at specified intervals of time from a specified depth below the surface without disturbing the suspension. The samples are dried and the residue is weighed. As the sizes of the particles are not uniform, the particles settle at different rates. The larger particles settle at a faster rate and fall below the pipette tip sooner than the smaller particles, thus each sample withdrawn has a lower concentration and contains particles of smaller diameter than the previous sample. From the weights of the dried samples the percentage of the initial suspension is calculated for particles having sizes smaller than the size calculated by Stoke's equation.

$$V_g = d^2 (P_p - P_1)/18\mu \times G$$

The process of sedimentation is employed in the operation of thickeners to settle out the solids in slurry and attain a clear overflow of the liquid. One assumption made in the operation of thickeners is that the material to be settled is in the form of flocs which are aggregate of finer materials sufficiently uniform in size and shape so that they settle at uniform velocities under conditions of hindered settling in the initial stages. Figure 4.4 shows a glass cylinder in which a batch settling operation is being conducted. The cylinder contains an initial uniform suspension, from this initial uniform suspension, any coarse material first falls to the bottom (layer E). Next a layer of settled solid (layer D) forms with a transition zone of partly thickened material above it C. The boundary between C and D is usually obscure and is marked by vertical channels through which water is escaping from the lower layers which are under compression. Next is a zone B of the material at the original concentration and finally a layer of clear water. The boundary between A and B is usually sharp. As thickening progresses, layer B and C ultimately disappear, but layer D may shrink

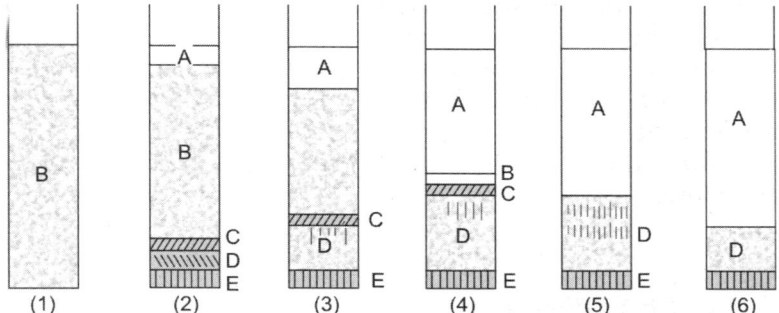

Fig. 4.4: Typical slurry-settling tests: A. Clear liquid; B. Slurry at original concentration; C. Transition zone; D. Thickened slurry in compression zone; E. Coarse solid

further because of compression. In such batch settling tests carried out at laboratory scale conditions and zone boundaries may vary with time.

Gravitational Sedimentation of Particles in a Liquid

Solids will settle in a liquid whose density is less than their own. At low concentration, Stokes' law will apply but in many practical instances the concentrations are too high.

In a cylinder in which a uniform suspension is allowed to settle, various quite well-defined **zones** appear as the settling proceeds. At the top is a zone of clear liquid. Below this is a zone of more or less constant composition, constant because of the uniform settling velocity of all sizes of particles. At the bottom of the cylinder is a zone of sediment, with the larger particles lower down. If the size range of the particles is wide, the zone of constant composition near the top will not occur and an extended zone of variable composition will replace it.

In a continuous thickener, with settling proceeding as the material flows through, and in which clarified liquid is being taken from the top and sludge from the bottom, these same zones occur. The minimum area necessary for a continuous thickener can be calculated by equating the rate of sedimentation in a particular zone to the counter-flow velocity of the rising fluid. In this case we have:

$$v_u = (F - L)\,(dw/dt)/AY$$

where, v_u is the upward velocity of the flow of the liquid, F is the mass ratio of liquid to solid in the feed, L is the mass ratio of liquid to solid in the underflow liquid, dw/dt is the mass rate of feed of the solids, Y is the density of the liquid and A is the settling area in the tank.

If the settling velocity of the particles is v, then $v_u = v$ and, therefore:

$$A = (F - L)(dw/dt)/v.$$

CYCLONE SEPARATOR

Cyclonic separation is a method of removing particulates from an air, gas or water stream, without the use of filters, through vortex separation (Fig. 4.5).

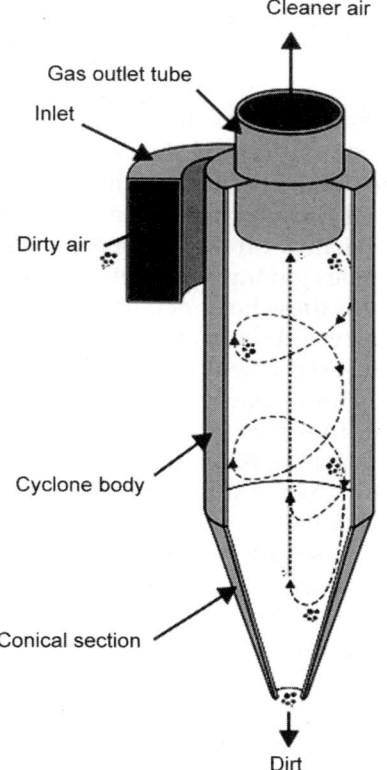

Fig. 4.5: Cyclone separator

Principle

In cyclone separator, the centrifugal force is used to separate solids from fluids. The separation depends not only on the particle size but also on particles. Hence, depending on the fluid velocity, the cyclone separator can be used to separate all types of particles to be carried through the fluids.

Construction and Working

Cyclones are made up of

1. Air inlet
2. Conical outer cylinder having a dirt bin.
3. Gas outlet tube

It consists of a cylindrical vessel with a conical base. In the upper part of the vessel is fitted with a tangential inlet and a fluid outlet and at the base it is fitted with solid outlet.

Dirty air comes in through the inlet. Cyclones are designed in such a way that they cause the incoming air to crash hard into the air already spinning inside the cyclone. The resulting very high turbulence breaks the heavier and lighter materials apart. The spinning air throws the heavier materials outward to the cyclone walls. Airflow on the cyclone walls is slowed by friction. Heavier particles get trapped in the slower moving air and gravity slowly pulls these heavier particles down. The cone on the bottom of the cyclone is angled just right to keep the airspeed constant to keep the heavier particles pressed tightly to the cyclone walls. These heavier particles continue to slide downward and eventually exit out a dust chute into the collection bin. The dust chute is sealed tightly to the bottom of the cyclone with no air leaks to stir up the collected dust. A full dust bin or bad air leak causes the cyclone to pump all right through with little or no separation. At the bottom of the cone there is a reversal point where the spinning air without these heavier particles moves in reverses direction and cleaned air then spirals up through the center of the cyclone then exits through the cyclone outlet.

The air entrance speed of a cyclone lies between 10 and 20 m/s, the most usual speed is approx. 16 m/s. The separation efficiency is given by the **Lappleis** formula which states that:

$$d_{50} = \sqrt{(9\mu b / 2\pi N \, \Gamma_i v_i)}$$

Here,

d_{50} = Particle sizes that with 50% outputs are broken away

b = Inlet width of the cyclone supply

N = Number of turn cycles in the cyclone

v_i = Inlet speed (m/s)

Γ_i = Specific mass of the dust particle (kg/m³)

μ = Viscosity of the gas (kg/m).

Advantages of a Cyclone Separator

- Simple in construction
- No moving components

- Little maintenance
- Low investment and functioning costs
- Less area is required

Disadvantages of a Cyclone Separator

- High pressure drop (0.5–2.5 kPa), depending on the construction version
- Low output for low particle diameter
- Emission of effluent at wet cyclone
- Erosion sensitive and constipation danger to the entrance
- Apparatus is noisy.

Uses

- Saw mills to remove sawdust from extracted air
- Cyclone separates are used to separate the suspension of a solid in a gas (air).
- Glass industry
- The foods industry
- Oil refineries to separate oils and gases
- Detritus combustion installations
- The chemical industry
- Melting processes in metallurgy
- Smaller cyclones are used to separate airborne particles for analysis.

ELUTRIATION METHODS

Elutriation, also known as **air classification**, is a process for separating lighter particles from heavier ones using a vertically-directed stream of gas or liquid (usually upwards). This method is profoundly used for particles with size (>1 µm) The smaller or lighter particles rise to the top (overflow) because their terminal velocities are lower than the velocity of the rising fluid. The terminal velocities of any particle in any media can be calculated using Stoke's law.

Stokes' Law

Stokes' law is a formula for determining the rate of sedimentation. It states that a particle moving through viscous liquid attains a constant velocity or sedimentation rate. The rate can be very slow for particles whose density is close to that of the liquid, for particles whose diameter is small, or where the viscosity is high. Replacing gravitational acceleration with the acceleration generated by a rotating centrifuge results in faster sedimentation. Centrifugal acceleration can be thousands of times greater than that of gravity, so the centrifugal sedimentation rate is thousands of times greater.

The following is the equation for Stokes' law of sedimentation:

$$V_g = d^2 (P_p - P_1)/18\mu \times G$$

where,

V_g = Sedimentation velocity

d = Particle diameter

P_p = Particle density

P_1 = Liquid density

G = Gravitational acceleration

μ = Viscosity of liquid

An air elutriator is a simple device which can separate particles into two or more groups.

Construction and Working

The size separation of powder is based on the low density of fine particles and high density of the coarse particles. Elutriating tank is used to separate the coarse and fine particles of powder after levitation, or paste made by levitation process is kept in an elutriating tank and mixed with large quantity of water. The solid particles are uniformly distributed in the liquid by stirring and then it is allowed to settle down. Depending on the density of solid particles, it will either settle down or remain suspended in water. The sample is withdrawn at different heights through the outlets. These are dried and thus the powders with various size fractions are collected as shown in the diagram.

The dry powder nowadays in elutriation process, the particles are suspended a moving fluid, generally water or air. The apparatus consists of a vertical column with an inlet near the bottom for suspension, outlets at the base for coarse particles

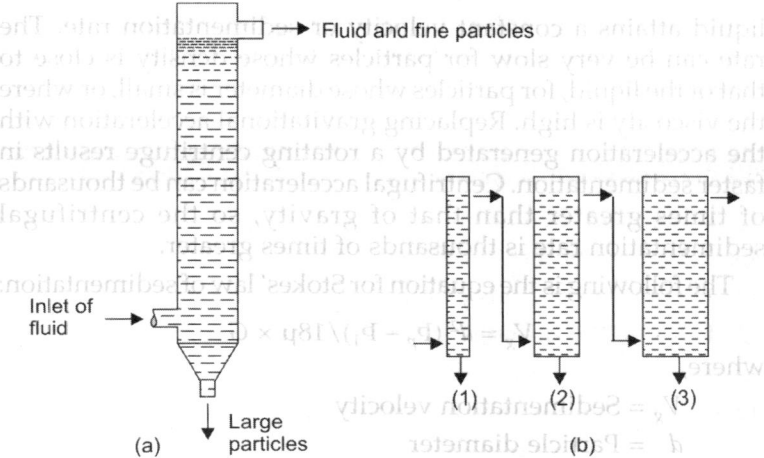

Fluid and fine particles

Inlet of fluid →

Large particles

(a)

(1)　(2)　(3)

(b)

Fig. 4.5: (a) Single stage elutriator, (b) Multi-stage elutriator

and an overflow near the top for fluid and fine particles. One column will give single separation into two fractions. If more than one fraction is required a number of tubes of increasing area of cross section can be connected in series. The velocity of the fluid decreases in succeeding tubes as the area of cross section increases, thus giving a number of fractions. These fractions are separated and dried.

Multiple elutriator: Flow rates can be increased to separate higher size ranges. Further size fractions may be collected if the overflow from the first tube is passed vertically upwards through a second tube of greater cross-section, and any number of such tubes can be arranged in series.

Advantages of Elutriation Method

1. The process is continuous.
2. Depending on the number of fractions required, the same number of tubes of different area of cross-section can be connected.
3. The separation is quick as compare to other methods of separation.
4. The apparatus is more compact than as that used in sedimentation methods.

The main disadvantage of this method is that the suspension of solid particles has to be diluted which may not be desired in certain cases.

PRACTISE QUESTIONS

Q. 1. Mention the various grades of powder.

Q. 2. Define the term "size separation".

Q. 3. What are various grades of coarse powder?

Q. 4. Name the different grades of fine powder.

Q. 5. Define the term "sieve number".

Q. 6. How size separation can be achieved by sedimentation?

Q. 7. Write short notes on:

a. Coarse powder

b. Fine powder

c. Very fine powder

Q. 8. Describe the process of sieving with the help of a neat and labeled diagram. What are the various methods of mechanical sieving?

Q. 9. Enlist the various standards for sieves. Give various factors affecting sieving.

Q. 10. Describe the process of sedimentation for size separation.

Q. 11. Give the principle, construction and working of cyclone separator with the help of a neat and labeled diagram.

Q. 12. Compare and contrast sedimentation and elutriation process for size separation.

Q. 13. What is elutriation? Give construction, working and advantages of elutriation process. How multiple elutriation is different from it?

OBJECTIVE TYPE QUESTIONS

Q. 1. Very fine powder is the one which ....

Q. 2. Sieve number indicates the number of mashes in a length of .... in each transverse direction parallel to the wires.

Q. 3. Equation for Stokes' law of sedimentation is ....
....

Q. 4. Match the following:

Type of powder	Sieve number (all particles must pass)
1. Coarse powder	a. 22
2. Moderately coarse powder	b. 10
3. Moderately fine powder	c. 44
4. Fine powder	d. 120
5. Very fine powder	e. 85

ANSWERS

1. All the particles must pass through sieve number 120.

2. 2.54 cm^2

3. $V_g = d^2 (\text{P}_p - \text{P}_1)/18\mu \times G$

4. 1-b, 2-a, 3-c, 4-e, 5-d.

5

Pharmaceutical Calculation

POSOLOGY

The term posology is derived from Greek word 'Poso' meaning "*how much*" and 'Logos' meaning "science". Hence, posology is a branch which deals with dose or quantity of drugs which can be administered to a patient to get desired pharmacological and therapeutic action. The dose cannot be fixed rigidly because there are so many factors which influence the doses. These factors are age, condition of the patient, severity of disease, tolerances both natural and acquired, idiosyncrasy, route of administration, type of formulation, drug interaction and rate of excretion.

Factors Affecting Dose

The optimum dose of a drug which produces the desired therapeutic effect varies from person to person. The dose range is usually based on the average requirement of an adult person depending upon his body weight, height, surface area and other parameters. The following are some factors which affect the dose:

Age: The pharmacokinetics **(ADME)** of many drugs changes with age. Hence, while determining the dose of a drug, the age of an individual is of a great importance. Children and old people need lesser amount of drug than the normal adult dose, because they are unable to excrete drugs to that extent as adults. In children, the various organs are less developed as compared to an adult one, especially in case of neonates special care is to be taken to dispense the drug.

Sex: Women do not always respond to action of drugs in same manner as man. Morphine and barbiturates may produce more excitement before sedation in women. Special care should be taken when drugs are administered during menstruation, pregnancy and lactation. The strong purgatives such as aloes should be avoided during menstruation. Similarly, the drugs which may stimulate the uterine smooth muscle, e.g. drastic purgatives, antimalarial drugs and ergot alkaloids are contraindicated during pregnancy. There are certain drugs which on administration to the mother are capable of crossing the placenta and affecting the fetus, e.g. alcohol, narcotics, barbiturates and non-narcotics, analgesics, etc. During lactation, the drugs like antihistaminic, morphine and tetracycline which are excreted in milk should be avoided or given very cautiously to the mothers who are breastfeeding the babies.

Body weight: The average dose is mentioned either in terms of mg per kg body weight or as a total single dose for an adult weighing between 50 o 100 kg. The dose expressed in this manner may not apply in case of obese patients, children and malnourished patients. It should be calculated according to body weight.

Route of administration: Intravenous doses of drugs are usually smaller than oral doses, because the drugs administered intravenously reaches the systemic circulation, i.e. the blood-stream directly. Due to this reason the onset of drug action is quick with intravenous route and this might enhance the chances of drug toxicity. The effectiveness of drug formulation is generally controlled by the route of administration. For example the same drug ranitidine can be given orally as well as parenteral route depending upon the type of severity of disease and condition of the patient.

Time of administration: The presence of food in the stomach delays absorption of drugs. The drugs are more rapidly absorbed from the empty stomach. So the amount of drug which is very effective when taken before meal may not be that much effective when taken during or after meals. Antacids are to be given before meals similarly enzymes preparation are to be given after meals.

Patient status: The personality and behavior of a patient may influence the effect of drug, especially the drug which is more intended for psychosomatic disorders. The females are more emotional than males and require lower dose of certain drugs. Inert dosage forms called placebos which resemble the actual medicament in physical properties are known to produce therapeutic benefit in diseases like angina pectoris and bronchial asthma.

Presence of disease: Drugs like barbiturates and chlorpromazine may produce unusually prolonged effects in patients liver cirrhosis. Streptomycin is excreted mainly by the kidney may prove toxic if the kidney of patient is not working properly. Similarly, patient suffering from liver ailment like jaundice than oral route is not preferred, drug is given parenteral so as to bypass liver. During fever a patient can tolerate high doses of antipyretics than a normal person.

Cumulative effect: The drugs which are slowly excreted may build up a sufficiently high concentration in the body and produce toxic symptoms, if it is repeatedly administered for a long time, e.g. digitalis, emetine and heavy metals .This occurs due to accumulative effect of the drug. The cumulative effects are usually produced by slow excretion, degradation and rapid absorption of drugs. Sometimes, a cumulative effect is desire in drugs like phenobarbitone in treatment of epilepsy.

Additive effect: When the total pharmacological action of two or more drugs administered together is equivalent to sum of their individual; pharmacological action, the phenomena is called as an additive effect. For example, combination of paracetamol and ibuprofen for analgesic effect.

Synergism: When two or more drugs used in combination form, their action is more than the individual effect of the drug. The phenomenon is called synergism. Synergism is very useful when desired therapeutic result needed is difficult to achieve with a single drug, e.g. procaine and adrenaline combination, increases the duration of action of procaine.

Idiosyncrasy (hypersensitivity reaction): An extraordinary response to a drug which is different from its characteristic pharmacological action is called idiosyncrasy. It is also called hypersensitivity reaction. There is difference in the term side effect and word idiosyncrasy, when a person is taking a drug then apart from its pharmacological action the drug is also causing some unwanted effects in the body these are called side effects while if a person is sensitive to a particular drug then on taking that drug allergic reactions takes place which can cause severe toxicity also these are termed as idiosyncrasy. For example, on taking a tablet of paracetamol some damage will occur to liver this is side effect of drug while if skin rashes appear than it is idiosyncrasy. Some persons are sensitive to penicillin and sulphonamides because they produce severe toxic symptoms.

Tachyphylaxis: It has been observed that when certain drugs are administered repeated at short intervals, the cell receptors get blocked up and pharmacological response to that particular drug is decreased. The decreased response cannot be reversed by increasing the dose. This phenomenon is known as tachyphylaxis or acute tolerance. For example, ephedrine when given in repeated dose at short intervals in treatment of bronchial asthma may produce very less response due to tachyphylaxis.

Pharmaceutical Calculations

To have a complete understanding of various types calculations, which are involved in dispensing, it is desirable that the pharmacist should have a thorough knowledge regarding weights and measures which are used in calculations.

There are two systems of weights and measures:
1. The imperial system
2. The metric system

1. The Imperial System

Measurement of weights in imperial system: Weight is a measure of the gravitational force acting on a body and is directly proportional to its mass. The imperial system is divided into two parts for the purpose of measurement of weight. These are:

• Avoirdupois system
• Apothecaries system

Avoirdupois system: In this system the pound is the standard unit for weighing and all measures of mass are derived from the Imperial Standard Pound (lb) (Table 5.1).

Table 5.1: Avoirdupois system for measurement

1 lb	= 16 oz (avoir)
1 lb	= 7000 grains
1 oz (avoir)	= 7000/16 grains
	= 437.5 grains

Apothecaries system: This system is also known as troy system. The grain is the standard weight in this system and all other weights are derived from it (Table 5.2).

Table 5.2: Avoirdupois system for measurement

20 grains	= 1 scruple (Э)
60 grains	= 1 drachm (3)
480 grains	= 1 ounces (3) (apothe)
8 drachms	= 1 ounces (apothe)
12 ounces	= 1 pound (lb)
5760 grains	= 1 pound (apothe)

Measurement of capacity in imperial system: The standard units for capacity is the same in both avoirdupois and apothecaries systems. The 'gallon' is the standard unit and all other measurements of capacity are derived it (Table 5.3).

Table 5.3: Measurement of capacity in imperial system

1 gallon (c)	= 160 fluid ounces
1/4th of a gallon	= 1 quart
1/8th of a gallon	= 1 pint (o)
1/160 of a gallon	= 1 fl ounce (3)
1/8th of a fl ounce	= 1 fl drachm (3)
1/60th of fl drachm	= 1 minim (m)
1 quart	= 40 fl ounces
1 pint	= 20 fl ounces
1 fl ounces	= 480 minims
1 fl drachm	= 60 minims

2. The Metric System

The metric system is used in Indian Pharmacopoeia for the measurement of weight and capacity. The metric system in India was implemented from 1st April, 1964 in pharmacy profession.

Measurement of weights in metric system: A 'kilogram' is the standard unit for measurement of weight and all other units are derived from it (Table 5.4).

Table 5.4: Measurement as per metric system

1 kilogram (kg)	= 1000 grams
1 hectogarm (hg)	= 100 grams
1 decagram (dag)	= 10 grams
1 decigram (dg)	= 10^{-1} gram
1 centigram (cg)	= 10^{-2} gram
1 miligram (mg)	= 10^{-3} gram
1 microgram (µg or mcg)	= 10^{-6} gram
1 gram (g)	= 1000 mg

Measurement of capacity: A 'liter' is the standard unit for measurement of capacity and all measurements of capacity are derived from it.

$$1 \text{ liter (lt)} = 1000 \text{ milliliters (ml)}$$

Conversion Tables

The Pharmacopoeia of India (IP) uses only metric system in formulae, but the prescriptions are still written in the imperial system by many an old time physician's. So a conversion (Tables 5.5 and 5.6) is used by pharmacists.

Table 5.5: Conversion tables

i. Weight measures

1 kilogram (kg)	= 2.2 lb (pound)
30 g	= 1 ounce (ℨ)
450 g	= 1 pound (avoir)
1 g	= 15 grains
60 mg	= 1 grain

ii. Capacity measures

1000 ml	= 1 quart
500 ml	= 1 pint
30 ml	= 1 fluid ounces
4 ml	= 1 fluid drachm
1 ml	= 15 minims
0.06 ml	= 1 minims

Table 5.6: Conversion table for domestic measures

Domestic measure	Metric system	Imperial system
1 drop	0.06 ml	1 minim
1 teaspoonful	4.00 ml	1 fluid drachm
1 dersert spoonful	8.00 ml	2 fluid drachm
1 tablespoonful	15.00 ml	4 fluid drachm
2 tablespoonful	30.00 ml	1 fluid ounce
1 wine glassful	60.00 ml	2 fluid ounce
1 teacupful	120.00 ml	4 fluid ounce
1 tumblerful	240.00 ml	8 fluid ounce

CALCULATION OF DOSES

The doses of a drug given represent the average maximum quantity of drugs which can be administered to an adult orally within 24 hours. When others routes of administration are followed, the dose is adjusted accordingly. The doses are also calculated in proportion to age, body weight and surface area of the patient.

1. Doses proportionate to age: There are a number of methods by which the dose for a child can be calculated from adult dose.

Young's formula

$$\text{Dose of a child} = \frac{\text{Age in years}}{\text{Age} + 12} \times \text{Adult dose}$$

The formula is used for calculating the doses of children less than 12 years of age.

Dilling's formula

$$\text{Dose of a child} = \frac{\text{Age in years}}{20} \times \text{Adult dose}$$

The formula is used for calculating the doses for children in between 4 and 20 years of age. This formula is considered better because it is easier and quick to calculate the dose.

Cowling's formula

$$\text{Dose of a child} = \frac{\text{Age in birthday}}{24} \times \text{Adult dose}$$

Fried's formula

$$\text{Dose of a child} = \frac{\text{Age in months}}{150} \times \text{Adult dose}$$

This formula is most useful for calculating the dose of kids less than 2 years of age.

Bastedo's formula

$$\text{Dose of a child} = \frac{\text{Age in yrs} + 3}{30} \times \text{Adult dose}$$

2. Doses proportionate to body weight: Clark's formula is used to calculate the dose for child according to body weight.

Clark's formula

$$\text{Dose of a child} = \frac{\text{Weight in pounds}}{150} \times \text{Adult dose}$$

3. Doses proportionate to surface area

$$\text{Dose of a child} = \frac{\text{Body surface area of child}}{\text{Body surface area of adult}} \times \text{Adult dose}$$

The calculation of child dose according to surface area is most satisfactory and appropriate rather than method based on age. The method is more complicated than method based on age. The body surface area is calculated from height and weight of the child. Table 5.7 shows the determination of children doses from adult doses on the basis of body surface area.

Table 5.7: Determination of children's dose from adult dose on the basis of body surface area

Sl. No.	Weight (kg)	Approx. surface area in square meters	Approx. percentage of adult dose
1	2	0.15	9
2	4	0.25	14
3	6	0.33	19
4	8	0.40	23
5	10	0.46	27
6	15	0.63	36
7	20	0.80	46
8	25	0.95	55
9	30	1.08	62
10	35	1.20	70
11	40	1.30	75
12	45	1.40	81
13	50	1.51	87
14	55	1.58	91

PRACTICE QUESTIONS

Q. 1. If the adult dose for a drug is 60 mg, what will be the dose (according to Young's formula) for:

a. 6 years child

b. 8 years child

Q. 2. If the adult dose for a drug is 200 mg, what will be the dose (according to Dilling's formula) for a:

a. 12 years child

b. 16 years child

Q. 3. If the adult dose for a drug is 100 mg, what will be the dose for a:

a. 6 months child

b. 24 months child

Q. 4. If the adult dose for a drug is 100 mg, what will be the dose (according to Bastedo's formula) for a:

a. 9 years child   b. 12 years child

Q. 5. If the adult dose for a drug is 100 mg, what will be the dose for a child weighing:

a. 24 lbs   b. 5 lbs

Q. 6. If the adult dose for a drug is 60 mg, what will be the dose for a child having surface area 1.2 m²?

Q. 7. The adult dose of a drug is 10 milligrams per kilogram of body weight. How many grams should be given to a patient weighing 220 lbs?

Q. 8. The adult dose of ampicillin suspension is 250 mg/5 ml four times daily. If a girl child is 3 ft 6 inches tall and weighs 93 lbs, how many milligrams will she receive for each dose?

Q. 9. If the usual dose of a drug is 200 milligrams, what would be the dose for an 8-year-old child who weighs 80 lbs?

ANSWERS

1. 20 mg, 16 mg

2. 120 mg, 160 mg

3. 4 mg, 16 mg

4. 40 mg, 50 mg

5. 16 mg, 10 mg

6. 41.6 mg

7. 1 gram

8. 166.18 mg or 3 ml

9. Fried's Rule: 128 mg, **Young's Rule:** 80 mg, **Clark's Rule:** 106.6 or 107 mg.

ENLARGING AND REDUCING RECIPES

Majority of the preparations made in a pharmacy are taken formulas that have been tested and are listed in the United States Pharmacopoeia/National Formulary (USP/NF) as official formulas. These formulas list the amount of each ingredient needed to formulate a specific quantity of preparation. Many a times it becomes necessary to reduce or enlarge a dose so as to formulate in a suitable dosage form.

1. Ratio and Quantity Method

Example: From the following formula below, calculate the amount of each ingredient needed to

Make 240 ml of Peppermint Spirit

Peppermint spirit	
Peppermint oil	100 ml
Peppermint powder	10 g
Alcohol	1000 ml (qs)

Solve first for the amount of peppermint oil needed
100 ml peppermint oil = X ml peppermint oil
1000 ml of spirit is 240 ml of spirit

Cross multiply: (1000) X = 100 (240)
1000 X = 24000
X = 24 ml of peppermint oil

Similarly, for the amount of peppermint powder needed
10 g peppermint powder = X g peppermint powder
1000 ml of spirit is 240 ml of spirit

Cross multiply: (1000) X = 10 (240)
1000 X = 2400
X = 2.4 g of peppermint powder

Since qs means to "add a sufficient quantity up to," take 2.4 g of peppermint powder add 24 ml of peppermint oil, and add alcohol to make 240 ml of final volume.

2. Conversion Factor Method

The conversion factor method is the easiest and therefore the most widely used method for reducing and enlarging the dose.

Example: From the following formula below calculate how much quantity of each ingredient will be required to prepare 240 ml of cocoa syrup?

Cocoa syrup	
Cocoa	180 g
Sucrose	600 g
Liquid glucose	180 ml
Glycerin	50 ml

Sodium chloride	2 g
Benzoic acid	1 g
Water	1000 ml (qs)

Calculation

The first step is to find the conversion factor, the 1000 ml of quantity is to be converted to 240 ml.

Hence, conversion factor = 240/1000 = 0.24

Now, multiply the conversion factor with the quantity of each ingredient in the original formula:

0.24 × 180 g = 43.2 g of cocoa

0.24 × 600 g = 144 g of sucrose

0.24 × 180 g = 43.2 g of liquid glucose

0.24 × 50 ml = 12 ml of glycerin

0.24 × 2 g = 0.48 g of NaCl

0.24 × 1.0 g = 0.24 g of benzoic acid

0.24 × qs 1,000 ml = 240 ml water (qs)

Hence, the following above quantity is to be taken mixed properly and finally the volume is to make up with 240 ml of water.

PRACTICE QUESTIONS

Q. 1. From the formula listed below, calculate the amount of each ingredient required to make 454 gm of baby powder.

Baby powder	
Boric acid	30 g
Zinc stearate	20 g
Talc	50 g

Q. 2. From the formula listed below calculate the amount of each ingredient required to make 12 ml of phenolated calamine lotion.

Phenolated calamine lotion	
Calamine lotion	990 ml
Liquid phenol	10 ml

Q. 3. From the formula listed below calculate the amount of each ingredient required to make 600 g of compound senna powder.

Compound senna powder	
Senna	18 g
Glycyrrhiza	23.6 g
Washed sulfur	8 g
Fennel oil	0.4 g
Sucrose	50 g

Q. 4. From the formula listed below calculate the amount of each ingredient required to make 10 ounces of pine tar ointment.

(**Note:** 1 ounce = 28.4 gm)

Pine tar ointment	
Yellow wax	150 g
Yellow ointment	350 g
Pine tar	500 g

ANSWERS

1. 136.2 g, 90.8 g, 227 g

2. 11.8 ml, 0.12 ml

3. 108 g, 141.6 g, 48 g, 2.4 g, 300 g

4. 42.6 g, 99.4 g, 142 g

ALLIGATION METHOD

When the calculation involves mixing of two similar preparations of different strength, to produce a preparation of intermediate strength, the alligation method is used. Alligation is a method used to solve problems that involve mixing two products of different strengths to form a product having a desired intermediate strength. Alligation is used to calculate (Fig. 5.1 and Flow chart 5.1):

a. The amount of diluent that must be added to a given amount of higher strength preparation to make a desired lower strength.

b. The amounts of active ingredient which must be added to a given amount of lower strength preparation to make a higher strength.

c. The amount of higher and lower strength preparations that must be combined to make a desired amount of an intermediate strength.

The method is recommended for the purpose of checking the calculations.

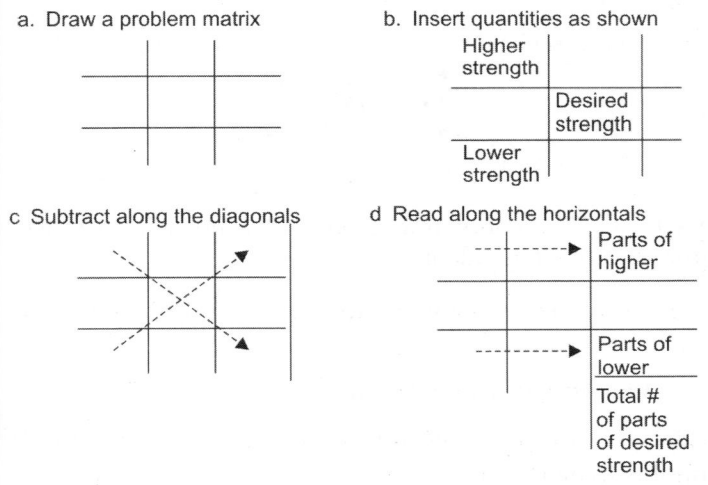

Fig. 5.1: Matrix showing percentage calculation method by alligation method

Flow chart 5.1: Matrix showing calculation of percentage of solution by alligation method

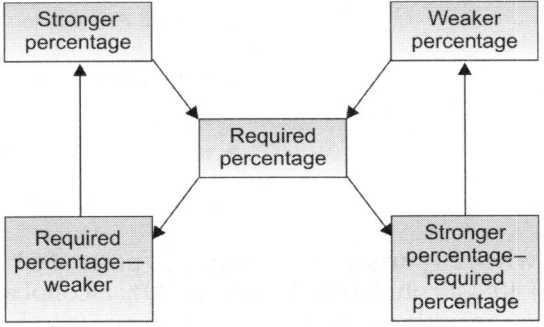

Example: *Calculate the volume of 95% alcohol required to prepare 300 ml of 70% alcohol by allegation method*

Calculation

Volume required = 300 ml

Percentage of alcohol required = 70

Percentage of alcohol used = 95

Using alligation method

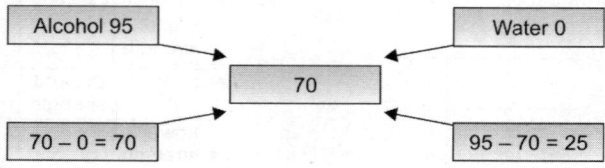

70 parts of 95% alcohol and 25 parts of water will produce the required percentage alcohol.

$$\text{Quantity of 95\% alcohol required} = \frac{300 \times 70}{95} = 221 \text{ ml}$$

$$\text{Quantity of water required} = \frac{300 \times 25}{9} = 79 \text{ ml.}$$

Hence, to produce 300 ml of 70% alcohol, 221 ml of 95% alcohol is to be taken.

Example: *Calculate the amount of 70%, 60%, 40% and 30% alcohol should be mixed to get 50% alcohol.*

Calculation: Using alligation method

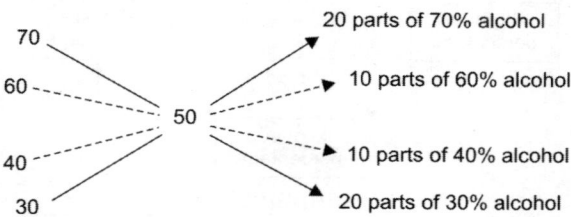

Hence, when 20 parts of 70% alcohol, 10 parts of 60% alcohol, 10 parts of 40% alcohol and 20 parts of 30% alcohol are mixed together, the resulting solution will produce 50% alcohol.

Example: Calculate the volume of each of 90%, 60%, 30% and water are required to produce 1000 ml of 40% alcohol

Calculation: Using alligation method

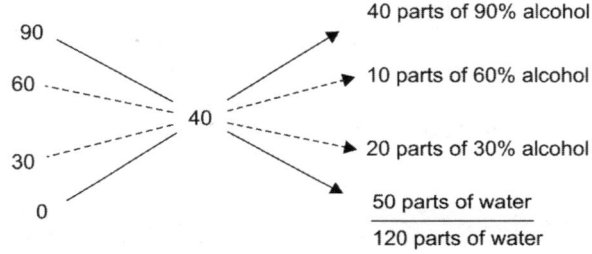

90

60

30

0

40

40 parts of 90% alcohol

10 parts of 60% alcohol

20 parts of 30% alcohol

$\dfrac{50 \text{ parts of water}}{120 \text{ parts of water}}$

When 40% parts of 90% alcohol, 10 parts of 60% alcohol, 20 parts of 30% alcohol and 50 parts of water are mixed together, the resulting solution will produce 40% alcohol.

1. Volume of 90% alcohol required
   = 120 parts: 1000 ml: 40 parts: v

   $$\text{Hence } v = \frac{1000 \times 40}{120} = \frac{40000}{120} = 333.3 \text{ ml}$$

2. Volume of 60% alcohol required
   =120 parts: 1000 ml: 10 parts: v

   $$\text{Hence } v = \frac{1000 \times 10}{120} = \frac{10000}{12} = 83.3 \text{ ml}$$

3. Volume of 30% alcohol required
   =120 parts: 1000 ml: 20 parts: v

   $$\text{Hence } v = \frac{1000 \times 20}{120} = \frac{20000}{120} = 166.6 \text{ ml}$$

4. Volume of water required = 1000 – 333.3 + 83.3 + 166.6
   $$= 573.2 \text{ ml}$$

PRACTICE QUESTIONS

Q. 1. In what proportion a solution containing 15% of a drug be mixed with 30% of same drug to get 20% mixture concentration?

Q. 2. What will be the % of alcohol obtained by mixing a solution containing 5 L of 25%, 1 L of 50% and 2 L of 95% alcohol?

Q. 3. In what proportion a solution containing 70% of a drug be mixed with 40% of same drug to get 50% mixture concentration?

Q. 4. In what proportion a solution containing 80%, 60%, 40%, 30% of a drug be mixed with to get 50% mixture concentration?

Q. 5. How much water is to be added to 700 ml of 92%, 850 ml of 86% and 600 ml of 26% alcohol to obtain a mixture of 20% strength?

ANSWERS

1. 5 parts of 30% and 10 parts of 15%.

2. 45.6%

3. 10 parts of 70% and 20 parts of 40%.

4. 10 : 20 : 30 : 10

5. 5504 ml.

PERCENTAGE PREPARATIONS

Many of the prescriptions received in the pharmacy have the amounts of active ingredients expressed as percentage strengths. The physician knows that each active ingredient, when given in certain percentage strength, gives the desired therapeutic effect. Instead of the physician calculating the amount of each ingredient needed for the prescription, he will simply indicate the percentage strength desired for each ingredient and expect the pharmacy to calculate the amount of each ingredient based on its percentage strength.

There are no percentage weights for a torsion balance or percentage graduations on a graduate. The percentage values on a prescription must be changed to amounts which can be weighed (grams) or to amounts, which can be measured (milliliters).

Types of Percent

The term percent means "parts per hundred" and is expressed in the following manner:

1. w/w percent: Weight/weight percent is defined as the number of grams in 100 grams (qs) of a solid preparation.

Example: A 5% (w/w) boric acid ointment would contain 5 gm of boric acid in each 100 grams (qs) of boric acid ointment.

Example: A 3% (w/w) vioform powder would contain 3 gm of vioform in every 100 gm (qs) of the vioform powder.

2. **w/v percent:** It is defined as the number of grams in 100 milliliters (qs) of solution.

Example: A 10% (w/v) potassium chloride (KCl) elixir would contain 10 gm of potassium chloride in every 100 milliliters (qs) of KCl elixir.

Example: A 5 percent (w/v) phenobarbital elixir would contain 5 gm of phenobarbital in every 100 milliliters (qs) of phenobarbital elixir.

3. **v/v percent:** It is defined as the number of milliliters in every 100 ml (qs) of solution.

Example: A 70% (v/v) alcoholic solution would contain 70 milliliters of alcohol in every 100 ml (qs) of solution.

Example: A 0.5% (v/v) glacial acetic acid solution would contain 0.5 milliliters of glacial acetic acid in each 100 milliliters (qs) of solution.

4. **v/w percent:** It is defined as the volume in milliliters of a substance in 100 gm (qs) of solution.

For example: A 10% (v/w) alcoholic solution would contain 10 milliliters of alcohol in every 100 gm (qs) of quantity sufficient solution.

When the type of percent is not stated, it is understood that dilutions are

1. For dry ingredient in a dry preparation is percent w/w
2. For dry ingredients in a liquid are percent w/v, and
3. For a liquid in liquid it is percent v/v.

ALCOHOL DILUTION

Dilute alcohols are prepared from 95% alcohol which contains 95 ml of ethyl alcohol and 5 ml of purified water quantity sufficient. When alcohol is mixed with water, the following changes take place:

1. Rise in temperature.
2. Contraction in volume.

3. There is turbid appearance in the solution, because solubility of air is more in alcohol than in water. When alcohol is diluted with water, minute bubbles of air get evolved and make turbid appearance. When alcohol is diluted with water, it is necessary to cool the mixture to about 20°C and then final volume is made up. The formula used is

Volume of stronger alcohol to be used =

$$\frac{\text{Volume required} \times \text{Percentage required}}{\text{Percentage used}}$$

Example: Calculate the amount of 95% alcohol required to prepare 200 ml of 45% alcohol.

Calculation

Volume required = 200 ml
Percentage of alcohol required = 45
Percentage of alcohol used = 95

By applying the formula

Volume of stronger alcohol to be used =

$$\frac{\text{Volume required} \times \text{Percentage required}}{\text{Percentage used}}$$
$$= \frac{200 \times 45}{95}$$
$$= 1800/19$$
$$= 94.7 \text{ ml}$$
$$\approx 95 \text{ ml (approx.)}$$

95 ml of 95% alcohol is diluted with water to produce 200 ml of 45% dilute alcohol.

Example: Calculate the volume of 95% alcohol required to produce 300 ml of 60% alcohol.

Calculation

Volume required = 300 ml
Percentage of alcohol required = 60
Percentage of alcohol used = 95

By applying formula

Volume of stronger alcohol to be used =

$$\frac{\text{Volume required} \times \text{Percentage required}}{\text{Percentage used}}$$

$$= \frac{300 \times 60}{95}$$
$$= 18000/95$$
$$= 189.47 \text{ ml}$$
$$\approx 190 \text{ ml (approx.)}$$

190 ml 95% alcohol is diluted with water to produce 300 ml 60% dilute alcohol.

Example: Calculte the quantity of sodium chloride required to prepare 400 ml of a 0.9% solution

Calculation

1% w/v solution means 1 gm in 100 ml

Hence, to prepare 400 ml (0.9%), sodium chloride required is

$$= \frac{0.9 \times 400}{100} \text{ gm, with solvent to produce 400 ml makes 0.9 \% w/v}$$

$$= 3.6 \text{ gm}$$

Hence 3.6 gm of sodium chloride is dissolved in water to produce 400 ml makes 0.9% w/v solution.

Example: Prepare 400 ml of a 5 per cent solution and from 2 L of solution having concentration 1 in 2,000.

Calculation

Strength of concentrate solution = 5%
Strength of dilute solution = 1 in 2000
$$= 1/2000$$
$$= 0.05\%$$

By applying formula

Digree of dilution = Strength of concentrate/strength of dilute solution

$$= 5/0.05$$
$$= 100 \text{ times}$$

Volume of the solution to be prepared = 2 L = 2,000 ml

Hence, dilute solution is obtained by diluting 2,000/100 = 20 ml of concentrate solution to 2 L.

Example: *Prepare 500 ml of a 1 in 400 solution from the 1 in 800 solution.*

Calculation

Strength of concentrate 1 in 800 =100/800 = 0.125%

Strength of dilute solution 1 in 4000 = 100/400 = 0.0025%

By applying formula

Degree of dilution = Strength of concentrate/strength of dilute solution

$$= 0.125/0.0025$$
$$= 50 \text{ times}$$

Volume of solution to be prepared = 500 ml

Hence, dilute solution is obtained by diluting 500/50 = 10 ml of 1 in 800 solution to 500 ml.

Dilution Method for Stock Preparations

In order to make formulation and preparation, the stock solution is diluted especially when the amount required is so small that it cannot be accurately weighed on a torsion balance. Since it is easier to measure an amount of stock solution than to weigh the ingredients.

Formulas Used

   a. Volumes and weights must be expressed in the same units.

   b. Concentrations must be expressed in the same units.

   c. *Formula:* $V_1 C_1 = V_2 C_2$

      V_1 = Volume of stock preparation

      C_1 = Concentration of stock preparation

      V_2 = Volume of desired preparation

      C_2 = Concentration of desired preparation

   d. *Formula:* $W_1 C_1 = W_2 C_2$

      W_1 = Weight of stock preparation

      C_1 = Concentration of stock preparation

      W_2 = Weight of desired preparation

      C_2 = Concentration of desired preparation

Example: How many milliliters of a 4% stock solution of potassium permanganate ($KMnO_4$) would be needed to compound 120 ml of 0.02% solution of $KMnO_4$?

Calculation

Using the formula

$$V1\ C1 = V2\ C2$$

Substituting the values

$$(X)\ (4\%) = (120\ ml)\ (0.02\%)$$

Checking the units and solving

a. Units of concentration are both %.

b. X will have the same units as the volume (i.e. ml)

$$4\ X = 2.4$$
$$X = 0.6\ ml$$

Example: How many grams of 15% zinc oxide ointment can be made from one pound of 20% zinc oxide ointment?

Calculation

Using the formula

$$W1\ C1 = W2\ C2$$

Substituting the values and solving

$$(X)\ (15\%) = (454\ g)\ (20\%)$$

Note: 1 lb = 454 gm.

$$15\ X = 9080\ X$$
$$= 605\ gm\ or\ 1.33\ lb$$

Example: How many milliliters of 10% povidone-iodine (betadine) solution would beneeded to make 2 L of a 1 : 2000 betadine solution?

Calculation

Using the formula

$$V1\ C1 = V2\ C2$$

Substituting the values

$$(X)\ (10\%) = (2\ L)\ (1/2000)$$

Checking the units and solving

a. Units of concentration of both are not in %.

b. X will have the same units as the volume (i.e. L)

Converting 10%, it will be 10/100

Now substituting and solving

$$(X).10/100 = (2). (1/2000)$$

$$X = 0.01 \text{ L or } 10 \text{ ml}$$

Example: How many milliliters of a 1 : 200 copper sulphate solution would be needed to make 2000 ml of a 1 : 4000 solution?

Calculation

$$V1\ C1 = V2\ C2$$

$$(X)\ (1/200) = (2000 \text{ ml})\ (1/4000)$$

$$20\ X = 2000 \text{ ml}$$

$$X = 100 \text{ ml}$$

PRACTICE QUESTIONS

Q. 1. How many milliliters of a 6% hydrogen peroxide solution would be needed to make 120 ml of 1% hydrogen peroxide solution?

Q. 2. How many milliliters of a 10% copper sulphate solution would be needed to make 60 ml of a 2% potassium copper sulphate solution?

Q. 3. How many milliliters of a 1 : 1000 cetrizine HCl solution are needed to make 90 ml of 1 : 5000 solution?

Q. 4. How many milliliters of a 1 : 50 stock solution should be used to prepare one liter of a 1 : 4000 solution?

Q. 5. How many milliliters of a 2.5% stock solution of a chemical should be used to make 5 L of a 1 : 1500 solution?

Q. 6. How many milliliters of a 1 : 200 stock solution should be used to make 120 ml of a 0.025% solution?

Q. 7. How many milliliters of a 1 : 50 stock solution should be used to make 1 L of a 0.02% solution?

Q. 8. How many milliliters of 10% (w/w) rose water can be made from 450 milliliters of 28% rose water?

Q. 9. How many gallons of 60% (v/v) alcohol can be made from 10 gallons of 95% (v/v) alcohol?

Q. 10. How many grams of 2% ammoniated mercury ointment can be made from 12.5 gm of 5% ammoniated mercury ointment?

Q. 11. How many grams of 10% betadine ointment can be made from 5 lbs. Of 15% betadine ointment?

Q. 12. How many grams of zinc oxide are needed to make 24 gm of a 4% (w/w) zinc oxide ointment?

Q. 13. How many milliliters of a 5% (w/v) boric acid solution can be made from 10 gm of boric acid?

Q. 14. How many milliliters of paraldehyde are needed to make 120 ml of a 20% (v/v) paraldehyde solution?

Q. 15. How many grams of ephedrine sulfate are needed to make 120 ml of a 2% (w/v) ephedrine sulfate solution?

Q. 16. How many grams of boric acid are needed to make 200 ml of a 5% (w/v) boric acid solution?

Q. 17. How many grams of zinc oxide are needed to make 120 gm of 10% zinc oxide paste?

Q. 18. How many grams of boric acid will be needed to make 400 gm of a 4% (w/w) ointment?

Q. 19. How many grams of strong silver protein (SSP) are required to make 250 ml of a 0.25% (w/v) solution?

Q. 20. How many grams of boric acid are there in 1 gallon of a 2% (w/v) boric acid solution?

Q. 21. If 10 gm of a chemical is dissolved in enough water to make the preparation measure one liter, what is the percentage strength of the solution?

Q. 22. How many milliliters of a 0.02% w/v solution can be made from 2.5 gm of a chemical?

Q. 23. Normal saline solution contains 0.9% w/v NaCl. How many grams of sodium chloride should be used to make 2 L of normal saline?

ANSWERS

1. 20 ml
2. 12 ml
3. 18 ml
4. 12.5 ml
5. 133 ml
6. 6 ml
7. 100 ml
8. 1260 gm
9. 15.3 gallons
10. 31.25 gm
11. 3405 gm or 7.5 lb
12. 0.96 gm
13. 200 ml
14. 24 ml
15. 2.4 gm
16. 10 gm
17. 12
18. 16 gm
19. 0.625 gm
20. 75.7 gm
21. 1%
22. 12,500 ml
23. 18 gm

ISOTONIC SOLUTIONS

Solution having the same osmotic pressure is called iso-osmotic. Osmosis is the movement of solvent through a membrane to equalize the concentration on both sides. The pressure required to allow for no transport of solvent across the membrane is called the osmotic pressure and obeys the relation (Fig. 5.2):

$$\pi = \frac{n_{solute}}{v_{solution}} RT = MRT$$

Isotonicity: If the concentrations of electrolytes are the same in the cell and surrounding fluid, the situation is balanced (homeostatic). The cell fluid volume remains the same.

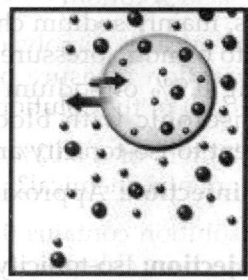

Fig. 5.2: Isotonic solution

Hypertonicity: The cell will shrink (crenation) by loss of its fluid to the surrounding hypertonic environment. High osmotic pressure of surrounding fluid pulls fluid out of the cell.

Hypotonicity: In a hypotonic environment, fluid will enter a cell and cause it to swell and burst. The inside of the cell has higher osmotic pressure than the surrounding fluid, so fluid is drawn into the cell (Fig. 5.3).

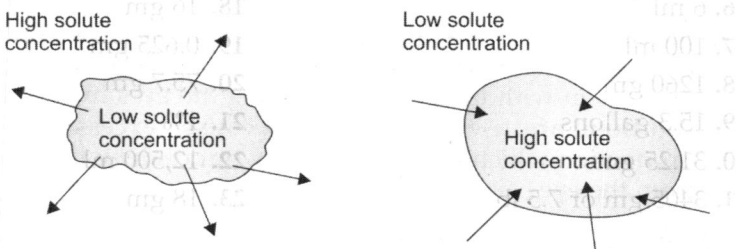

Fig. 5.3: Hypertonic solution and hypotonic solution

Both hypertonicity and hypotonicity in the extracellular fluids will destroy cells. Need isotonicity for cell homeostasis, for balance. To determine whether or not a solution is isotonic with erythrocytes, it is necessary to determine the concentration of the solute at which the cells retain their normal size and shape. The parenteral solution and ophthalmic solutions need adjustment to iso-osmoticity and iso-tonicity.

The solutions which are not having the same osmotic pressure are called 'paratonic'. Which comparing a solution with the one of known osmotic pressure, those which exert a greater pressure are called 'hypertonic, blood make the contains 0.88% of inorganic salts, mainly sodium chloride, which make the main contribution to osmotic pressure.

A solution cotaining 0.9% of sodium chloride and 5.4% dextrose solution is isotonic with blood plasma general principles for adjustment to iso-tonicity are:

1. **Solutions for I/V injection:** Approximate iso-tonicity is always desirable.

2. **Solution for S/C injection:** Iso-tonicity is required but not essential' since they are injected into fatty tissues.

3. **Solutions for I/M injection:** The aqueous solutions should be slightly hypertonic to promote rapid absorption.

4. **Solution for intrathecal injection:** These must be isotonic, because the volume of CSF is only 60 to 80 ml. Hence, a small volume of a para-tonic solution will disturb the osmotic pressure may cause vomiting and other side-effects.

5. **Solution used for nasal drops:** Isotonicity is needed, since Para-tonic solution may cause irritation.

6. **Solution used as eye drops and eye lotion:** Eye lotion should be isotonic with lacrimal secretion, since a large volume is brought in with the eye. For washing the eyes hypertonic solutions are used because they causes excessive tear production which helps in draining out of dirty materials from the eye.

Calculation Based on Isotonicity

1. Based on freezing point method

   Percentage w/v of adjusting substance needed

   $$= 0.52 - a/b$$

   here a = Freezing point of the unadjusted solution

   b = Freezing point of a 1% w/v of adjusting substance.

2. Based on molecular concentration

   Percentage w/v of adjusting substance required

   $$= 0.03 \, M/N$$

Example: Calculate the amount of procaine hydrochloride which will give a solution iso-osmotic with blood plasma (The freezing point of 1% w/v solution of procaine hydrochloride is −0.122°C.)

Calculation: By applying the formula

Percentage w/v of adjusting substance needed = 0.52 − a/b

$$= 0.52 - 0.0$$

$$= \frac{0.52 - 0.0}{0.122}$$

$$= 4.2\% \, w/v$$

Note: a = 0 (freezing point of unadjusted solution is to be taken zero when not given)

Example: *Calculate the amount of sodium chloride required to make 1% solution of boric acid iso-osmotic with blood plasma. (The freezing point of 1% w/v solution of boric acid is –0.288°C and the freezing point of 1% w/v solution of sodium chloride is –0.576°C.)*

Calculation: By applying the formula

Percentage w/v of adjusting substance needed = 0.52 – a/b

$$= \frac{0.52 - 0.288}{0.576}$$

$$= 0.39\% \text{ w/v}$$

Example: *Calculate the amount of sodium chloride required to make 1.5% solution of boric acid iso-osmotic with blood plasma. (The freezing point of 1% w/v solution of boric acid is –0.288°C and the freezing point of 1% w/v solution of sodium chloride is –0.576°C.)*

Calculation: By applying the formula
Percentage w/v of adjusting substance needed

$$= 0.52 - a/b$$

$$= \frac{0.52 - (0.288 \times 1.5)}{0.576}$$

$$= 0.15\% \text{ w/v}$$

PRACTICE QUESTIONS

Q. 1. What concentration of cocaine hydrochloride will give solution iso-osmotic with blood plasma? The freezing point of 1% w/v solution of cocaine hydrochloride is –0.09°C.

Q. 2. What concentration of lignocaine hydrochloride will give solution iso-osmotic with blood plasma? The freezing point of 1% w/v solution of cocaine hydrochloride is –0.09°C.

Q. 3. What concentration of sodium chloride is required to make 1% solution of adrenaline iso-osmotic with blood plasma? The freezing point of 1% w/v solution of adrenaline is –0.09°C and the freezing point of 1% w/v solution of sodium chloride is –0.576°C.

Q. 4. What concentration of sodium chloride is required to make 1.5% solution of procaine hydrochloride iso-osmotic with blood plasma? The freezing point of 1% w/v solution of procaine hydrochloride is $-0.122°C$ and the freezing point of 1% w/v solution of sodium chloride is $-0.576°C$.

ANSWERS

1. 5.77% w/v   **2.** 5.71% w/v

3. 0.732% w/v   **4.** 0.585% w/v

PROOF SPIRIT

For excise purpose, the strength of alcoholic preparations are indicated by degrees, **"over proof"** or **"under proof"**. Proof spirit is that mixture of alcohol and water which at 51°F weighs 12/13th of an equal volume of water.

In India, 57.1 volume of ethyl alcohol is considered to be equal to 100 volumes of proof spirit. This means that any alcoholic solution which contains 57.1% v/v alcohol is a proof spirit which is said to be 100 proof. Hence, strength above proof strength is expressed as over proof (OP) and any strength below proof strength is expressed as under proof (UP).

For excise purpose in India the proof alcohol is calculated in terms of rupees per litre of proof alcohol. So any percentage volume in volume of alcohol can be converted into proof strength and *vice versa* by using the following method:

1. Multiply the percentage strength of alcohol by 1.753 and subtracting 100 from it.
2. If the result is positive, it is known as over proof (OP)
3. If the result is negative, it is known as under proof (UP).

The value 1.753 used in the formula is calculated as

57.1 volumes of ethyl alcohol = 100 volume of proof spirit

1 volume of ethyl alcohol = 100/57.1 = 1.753 volume of proof spirit .

Example: *Find strength of 85% v/v alcohol in terms of proof spirit.*

Solution: By applying the formula:

Percentage strength of alcohol × 1.753 – 100

$$= 85 \times 1.753 - 100$$
$$= 149 - 100 = +49 \qquad \text{i.e. } 49° \text{ OP.}$$

Example: Find strength of 60% v/v alcohol in terms of proof spirit.

Solution: By applying the formula:

Percentage strength of alcohol $\times$ 1.753 – 100

$$= 60 \times 1.753 - 100$$
$$= 105.2 - 100 = +5.2. \qquad \text{i.e. } 5.2° \text{ OP}$$

Example: Find strength of 45% v/v alcohol in terms of proof spirit.

Solution: By applying the formula:

Percentage strength of alcohol $\times$ 1.753 – 100

$$= 45 \times 1.753 - 100$$
$$= 78.9 - 100 = -21.1 \qquad \text{i.e. } 21.1° \text{ UP}$$

Example: Calculate the strength of 30° OP and 40° UP

Solution: By applying the formula:

30° over proof means 100 + 30 = 130

Alcohol strength = 130/1.753 = 74.15% v/v

(i.e. 74.15% solution diluted to 100 ml qs will give 30° OP solution.)

40° under proof means 100–40 = 60

Alcohol strength = 60/1.753 = 34.23% v/v

(i.e. 34.23% solution diluted to 100 ml qs will give 40° UP solution.)

Example: How many proof gallons are there in 5 of 65%v/v alcohol?

Calculation: Applying the formula:

Value in proof = % strength of alcohol $\times$ 1.753 – 100

$$= 65 \times 1.753 - 100$$
$$= 113.9 - 100$$
$$= +13.9$$
$$= 13.9° \text{ OP}$$

It means

100 gallons of 65 % v/v alcohol = 113.9 units of proof spirit

1 gallon of 65% v/v alcohol = 113.9/100

Hence, 5 gallons of 65% v/v alcohol $= \dfrac{113.9 \times 3}{100}$

$$= 5.7 \text{ gallons of proof spirit}$$

Hence, 5 gallons of 65% v/v alcohol are equivalent to 5.7 gallons of proof spirit.

PRACTICE QUESTIONS

Q. 1. Convert the following degrees of proof into percentage under proof:
a. 12.1° UP
b. 21.5° UP
c. 54.8° UP

Q. 2. Convert the following degrees of proof into percentage over proof:
a. 44.6° OP
b. 35.3° OP
c. 18.4° OP

Q. 3. How many proof gallons are there in 5 of 70% v/v alcohol?

ANSWERS

1. a-50.14%, b-44.78%, c-25.78%
2. a-82.49%, b-77.18%, c-67.54%
3. 6.13 gallon

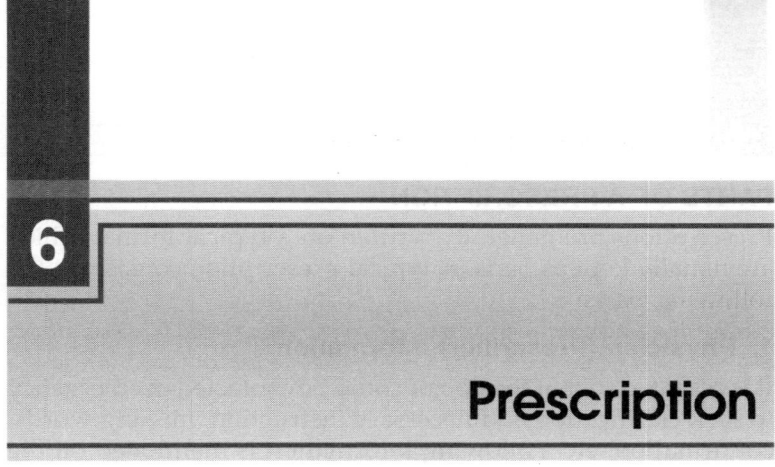

6

Prescription

"A medical prescription is an order (often in written form) by a qualified health care professional to a **pharmacist** or other therapist for a treatment to be provided to their **patient**".

A prescription is a legal document which not only instructs in the preparation and provision of the medicine or device but indicates the prescriber takes responsibility for the clinical care of the patient and the outcomes that may or may not be achieved.

R_x

There are various theories about the origin of this symbol—some note its similarity to the **Eye of horus,** others to the ancient symbol for **Jupiter,** both gods whose protection may have been sought in medical contexts. Alternatively, it may be intended as an abbreviation of the **Latin** "recipe", the imperative form of "recipere", "to take", and it is quite possible that more than one of these factors influenced its form. Literally, "Recipe" means simply "Take ...." and when a doctor writes a prescription beginning with "R_x", he or she is completing the command. This was probably originally directed at the pharmacist who needed to take a certain amount of each ingredient to compound the medicine, rather than at the patient who must "take" the medicine, in the sense of consuming it. The word "prescription" can be decomposed into "pre" and "script" and literally means, "to write before" a drug.

PARTS OF A PRESCRIPTION

Prescriptions are generally written on a typical format which are usually kept as pads. A typical prescription consists of the following parts:

1. Physician (Prescriber) Information

It is essential so that the doctor could be contacted in emergency to seek clarification and necessary instruction, missing words, confirmation, etc. Following information is mentioned on the prescription:

i. Doctor's name, designation and registration number
ii. Address with phone number and e-mail.
iii. Date of issue of prescription.
iv. Prescription number (required when calling the pharmacy for a refill or for medical claim purposes).

2. Patient Information

The name, address, age and sex of the patient help in identifying the prescription. Date of prescribing and date(s) of presentation for filling are necessary for keeping accurate records and ascertaining the needs of the patient. Age and sex of the patient, if mentioned, help the pharmacist to check the pre-scribed dose(s) of the medication.

3. Superscription

The superscription which consists of the heading where the symbol R_x (an abbreviation for recipe, the Latin for 'take thou' or 'you take' is found. R_x symbol comes before the inscription. The sign at the foot of the letter R is believed to represent the sign of Jupiter, the God of healing. Some historians believe that the symbol R_x originated from the sign of Jupiter.

4. Inscription

The inscription (body of prescription) comprises an important part of prescription containing:

i. Name(s) of drug(s) and their quantities,
ii. Other chief ingredients of the prescription with quantity,
iii. Instruction regarding dosage form like tablet, capsule, suspension, mixture, etc. and
iv. Dose and quantity of prescription

5. Subscription

The subscription gives specific directions for the pharmacist on how to compound the medication. Most of direction is usually expressed in contracted Latin or in the form of abbreviation. Instructions for preparation are also given such as: 'make a mixture', 'mix and make 10 tablets', or 'dispense 10 tablets'.

6. Signatura

The signatura which gives instructions to the patient. These instructions are preceded by abbreviation 'Sig.' from the Latin, meaning 'mark.' The signatura should always be written in English; however, physicians continue to insert Latin abbreviations, e.g.' 1 cap t.i.d. pc' which the pharmacist translates into English as 'take one capsule three times daily after meals'. It may also contain special instructions, warnings, followed by the signature of the prescriber.

7. Renewal

The number of times a prescription is to be repeated, is written by the physician under renewal instructions.

8. Signature

Finally the prescription must bear the signature of the prescriber to impart it the legal validity.

9. Other Important Instructions

a. **Qty:** "Quantity" or how much is in the package.

b. **Mfg:** "Manufacturer" or who makes the medication.

c. **Expiry date:** When the drug is going to expire.

d. **Take complete/full course:** Means that patient should finish taking the entire contents of the prescription even if feeling better especially patient taking antibiotics. This is to avoid recurrence of infection and development of resistance.

e. **Take with/without food:** Means whether the medication is to be taken after a meal or empty stomach. Some medications work better when the stomach is full while some medications work better when the stomach is empty.

f. Take four times a day: Means to take the medication four times in 24 hours with equal spacing of time. It is different than 'take every four hours'. If any confusion occurs when to give the medications, one should consult doctor or pharmacist. Most medications do not have to be precisely timed to be effective, but some do.

g. Take as needed as symptoms persist: Means the medication can be taken when symptoms are present, without consulting the prescriber.

   i. The package may also have bright colored warning labels with additional information. The following examples are:

   i. Safe storage instructions, such as 'keep refrigerated'.

   ii. Instructions for use, such as 'shake well before use'.

   iii. Possible side effects, such as 'may cause drowsiness'.

The use of Latin in prescription writing is traditional (Fig. 6.1). Although teaching of Latin has slowly gone out of the curricula of medicine and pharmacy, some of the words

AGARWAL NURSING HOME		
Khatghar, Quila, Bareilly Ph: 0581–2514560		
		Date: 28-2-08
Name: Mr. Ashish Agarwal	Age: 19 Years	Sex: Male
Address: 51, Parvez Coloney, Bareilly.		
R_x (Superscription)		
(Inscription)	Sodium bicarbonate Compound tincture of cardamon Simple syrup Water qs	3 gm 2 ml 6 ml 90 ml
Fiat mistura (subscription)		
Sig. Cochlear magnum ter in die post cibos sumenda (signatura)		
Refill:	Sd/– Dr. S.K. Agarwal M.B.B.S., M.D. Regd. No. 14328	

Fig. 6.1: Typical prescription

and abbreviations have very deep roots and physicians still use them frequently. In earlier days, a prescription was a secret between the physician and the pharmacist and a mystery for the patient. With the increasing awareness about drugs no secrecy is now warranted. As such the patient has a right to know what medication has been prescribed and his interest is protected under the Consumer Protection Act.

HANDLING OF PRESCRIPTION

The following procedure should be adopted by the pharmacist while handling the prescription for compounding and dispensing:

1. Receiving
2. Reading and checking
3. Collecting and weighing the materials
4. Compounding, labeling and packaging

1. **Receiving:** The prescription should be received from the patient by the pharmacist himself. While receiving a prescription, a pharmacist should not change his facial expression which gives an impression to the patient that he is surprised or confused after seeing the prescription.

2. **Reading and checking:** On receiving a prescription, always check it that it is written in a proper format, i.e. doctor's pad or OPD slip of the hospital/nursing home and is duly signed by the prescriber along with date. A prescription should always be screened behind the counter. In case of any difficulty in reading or any doubt regarding the prescription ingredients or directions, the pharmacist should consult the other pharmacist or the prescriber. But under no circumstance patient should come to know about it. Pharmacist should never guess about the meaning of any illegal or confused word. It may lead to serious consequences.

Sometimes prescription is received on telephone by senior pharmacist. In such case, after taking down the prescription, it should be verified by repeating it on phone to the prescriber, It is very important because nowadays, the number of drugs with almost the same pronunciation and spelling are available in the market.

For example:

Acidin (R)	Apidin (R)
Prednisone	Prednisolone
Digoxin	Digitoxin
Althrocin	Eltroxin

It there is any omission of any important particulars, such as the dose, the prescriber should be contacted.

3. **Collecting and weighing the material:** Before compounding the prescription, all the materials required for it, should be collected on the left hand side of the balance. After weighing the material it should be shifted to right hand side of the balance. This gives a check of ingredients which have been weighed. While compounding, the label of every stock should be read at least three times in order to avoid any error:

   a. When taken from the shelf or drawer.

   b. When the contents are removed for weighing and measuring.

   c. When the containers are returned back to their proper place.

4. **Compounding, labelling and packaging:** Compounding should be carried out in a neat place. All the equipment, etc. required should be thoroughly cleaned and dried. Only one prescription should be compounded at one time. All the ingredients should be compounded according to the directions of the prescriber or according to pharmaceutical art. The compounded medicaments should be filled in suitable containers depending on their quantity and use. The filled containers are suitably labelled. White plain paper of good quality should be used for labelling the containers. The size of the label should be proportional to the size of the container which is written or typed, giving all the desired information. The label should be fixed with a good quality of adhesive, almost in the centre leaving equal space from the bottom and top of the container. The container is polished so as to remove the fingerprints. While delivering the prescription to the patient, the pharmacist should

explain the mode of administration, direction for use, and storage.

MODERN METHODS OF PRESCRIBING

Nowadays, the majority of the drugs are available in the market as ready-made formulations manufactured by different pharmaceutical companies. There is no need to dispense the drugs by the pharmacist. In the present days, the role of pharmacist is to hand over the ready-made preparations to the patients and provide advice if demanded regarding its mode of administration, dose schedule, drug interactions and adverse reactions, etc. The practice of writing long, complicated prescriptions containing several ingredients, adjuvants, or vehicles is not required.

In the present day set up, the writing of prescription is more significant. The prescription should be precise, accurate, clear and easily readable. As far as possible, the Latin terms should be avoided. In olden days the Latin language was used to conceal certain facts from the patient. But nowadays, the prescriptions are written in English language and dose is prescribed in metric system for the convenience of the patients.

The drugs should be prescribed by their official (generic) name and not by proprietary or trade name. There are certain advantages and disadvantages of prescribing the drugs by proprietary names, which are as under:

Advantages

1. It is easy to remember proprietary names because they are very catchy, e.g. librium (chlordiazepoxide), calmpose (diazepam), and crocin (paracetamol).

2. It is easy to communicate with the patient.

3. The continuity can be maintained by prescribing the same proprietary name every time.

4. The bioavailability of drugs changed with the change of adjuvants used in drug formulations manufactured by different manufacturers. So, only those proprietary drugs can be prescribed which have a better bioavailability.

Disadvantages

1. It is cheaper to prescribe the drugs by their official names.
2. It becomes difficult for a pharmacist to dispense the substitute of the drug which is available in the stock.

There are four types of prescriptions which are generally received by the retail drug store:

a. Prescription in general practice
b. Private prescriptions
c. Hospital prescriptions meant for 'out patients'
d. Hospital prescriptions meant for 'in patients'

A typical modern prescription is shown below (Fig. 6.2).

AGARWAL NURSING HOME Khatghar, Bareilly Tel.: 0581-2514530 Mob: 09259082272	
	Date: 20-1-08
Name: Mrs. Tanvi Agarwal Age: 21 Yrs	Sex: Female
Address: 55, Parvez Coloney, Bareilly R_x Capsule: Ampicillin 500 mg Dispense 20 capsules. One capsule to be taken with water four times a day for five days.	
Refill:	Sd/– Dr. Abhinav Agarwal M.B.B.S., M.D. Regd. No. 0122345

Fig. 6.2: Modern form of prescription

CARE REQUIRED IN DISPENSING PRESCRIPTION

Following precautions should be taken while dispensing a prescription.

1. The pharmacist should keep the prescription himself. The prescription should be taken while taking out the medicine from the shelf. It will serve as a constant reminder of the

name and strength of the preparation required and help to avoid mistake.

2. Always check the dispensing balance before weighing the ingredients which are required during dispensing.

3. Replace containers of stock preparations or drugs in their proper position after use.

4. Keep the label in upper position during weighing solid ingredients, especially the potent drugs such as morphine hydrochloride to serve as a constant reminder that the correct drug is being used.

5. When pouring or measuring the liquid ingredients, keep the label upward in order to prevent surplus running down of the bottle and staining the label.

6. Care should be taken to keep the dispensing balance clean. The powder should be transferred from the stock container by using a clean spatula. The scale pan should be cleaned immediately after use.

7. Medicines which are used externally such a lotions, liniments, paints, etc. should be supplied in vertically fluted or ribbed bottles in order to distinguish it by touch. They must be labeled in red or against a red background. **"For external use only"**.

8. Before handing over the medicine to the patient, again check that the correct preparation, in the correct strength, has been supplied and correct direction has been stated on the label.

SOURCES OF ERROR IN PRESCRIPTION

1. **Abbreviation:** Abbreviation presents a problem in understanding parts of the prescription order. Extreme care should be taken by a pharmacist in interpreting the abbreviations. Pharmacist should not guess at the meaning of an ambiguous abbreviation, e.g. to dispense Achromycin for "Achro" may cause difficulty when the intention of the prescriber is to dispense Achrostatin. The abbreviation "SSKT" represents the use of a shorthand for saturated solution and chemical symbols for potassium iodide.

2. Name of the drug: There are certain drugs whose names look or sound-like those of other drugs. Some of the examples of such drugs are as under:

Digitoxin	Digoxin
Prednisone	Prednisolone
Indocin	Lincocin
Doridon	Doxidan
Pabalate	Robalate
Ananase	Orinase

Names of the pharmaceutical products have been changed on certain occasion due to the possible confusion with the name of the other product, e.g. the name of potassium supplement was changed from kalyum to kolyum because of the possible confusion of the former designation with valium.

3. Strength of the preparation: The strength of the preparation should be stated by the prescriber. It is essential when various strengths of a product are available in the market. For example, it will be a wrong decision on the part of a pharmacist to dispense paracetamol tablet 500 mg when prescription for paracetamol tablet is received with no specific strength.

4. Dosage form of the drug prescribed: Many medicines are available in more than one dosage form, e.g. liquid, tablet, capsule and suppository. The pharmaceutical form of the product should be written on the prescription in order to avoid ambiguity.

5. Dose: Unusually high or low doses should be discussed with the prescriber. Pediatric dosage may present a problem. So, pharmacist should consult pediatric posology to avoid any error. Sometimes a reasonable dose is administered too frequently, e.g. a prescription for sustained release formulation to be administered after very four hours should be thoroughly checked because such dosage forms are usually administered only two or three times a day.

6. Instructions for the patient: The instructions for the patient which are given in the prescription may be incomplete or omitted. The quantity of the drug to be taken, the frequency and timing of administration, and route of administration should be clearly given in the prescription so as to avoid any confusion.

7. **Incompatibilities:** It is essential to check that there are no pharmaceutical or therapeutic incompatibilities in a prescribed preparation and that different medicines prescribed for the same patient do not interact with each other to produce any harm to the patient. Certain antibiotics should not be given with meals since it significantly decreases the absorption of the drug.

LEGALITY OF PRESCRIPTION

Prescriptions, when handwritten, are notorious for being often illegible (5% according to an Irish study. Contrary to popular belief, pharmacists do not have special deciphering skills. When in doubt, they call the doctor. At other times, even though some of the individual letters are illegible, the position of the legible letters and length of the word is sufficient to distinguish the medication based on the knowledge of the pharmacist.

Writing Good Prescription

Following are some tips for writing good prescription:

1. Careful use of decimal points to avoid ambiguity.
2. Avoid unnecessary decimal points: 5 ml instead of 5.0 ml to avoid possible misinterpretation of 5.0 = 50
3. Always zero prefix decimals, e.g. 0.5 instead of .5 to avoid misinterpretation with .5 = 5.
4. Avoid decimals altogether by changing the units: 0.5 gm = 500 mg.
5. "ml" is used instead of "**cc**" or "**cm³**" even though they are technically equivalent.
6. Quantities can be given directly or implied by the frequency and duration of the direction.
7. Where possible, usage directions should specify times (7 am, 3 pm, 11 pm) rather than simply frequency (3 times a day) and especially relationship to meals for orally consumed medication.

Partial list of prescription abbreviations

Abbreviation	Latin	Meaning
aa	ana	of each
ad	Ad	up to
a.c.	ante cibum	before meals
a.d.	aurio dextra	right ear
ad lib.	Ad libitum	use as much as one desires; freely
admov.	admove	apply
agit	agita	stir/shake
alt. h.	alternis horis	every other hour
a.m.	ante meridiem	before noon morning,
amp		ampule
amt		amount
aq	aqua	water
a.l., a.s.	aurio laeva, aurio sinister	left ear
A.T.C.		around the clock
a.u.	auris utrae	both ears
bis	bis	twice
b.i.d.	bis in die	twice daily
B.M.		bowel movement
bol.	bolus	as a large single dose (usually intravenously)
B.S.		blood sugar
B.S.A		body surface areas
cap., caps.	capsula	capsule
c	cum	with (usually written with a bar on top of the "c")
c	cibos	food
cc	cum cibos	with food, (but also cubic centimeter)
cf		with food
comp.		compound
cr., crm		cream
D5W		dextrose 5% solution (sometimes written as D5W)
D5NS		dextrose 5% in normal saline (0.9%)
D.A.W.		dispense as written

dc, D/C,		disc discontinue
dieb. alt.	diebus alternis	every other day
dil.		dilute
disp.		dispense
div.		divide
d.t.d.	dentur tales doses	give of such doses
D.W.		distilled water
elix.		elixir
e.m.p.	Ex modo prescripto	asdirected
emuls.	emulsum	emulsion
et	Et	and
ex aq	Ex aqua	in water
fl., fld.		fluid
ft.	fiat	make; let it be made
gm		gram
gr		grain
gtt(s)	gutta(e)	drop(s)
H		hypodermic
h, hr	hora	hour
h.s.	hora somni	at bedtime
ID		intradermal
IM		intramuscular (with respect to injections)
inj.	injectio	injection
IP		intraperitoneal
IV		intravenous
IVP		intravenous push
IVPB		intravenous piggyback
L.A.S.		label as such
LCD		coal tar solution
lin	linimentum	liniment
liq	liquor	solution
lot.		lotion
M.	misce	mix
m, min	minimum	a minimum
mcg		microgram

mEq		milliequivalent
mg		milligram
mist.	mistura	mix
mitte	mitte	send
ml		milliliter
nebul	nebula	a spray
N.M.T.		not more than
noct.	nocte	at night
non rep.	non repetatur	no repeats
NS		normal saline (0.9%)
1/2NS		half normal saline (0.45%)
N.T.E.		not to exceed
o_2		both eyes, sometimes written as O_2
o.d.	oculus dexter	right eye
o.s.	oculus sinister	left eye
o.u.	oculus uterque	both eyes
oz		ounce
per	per	by or through
p.c.	post cibum	after meals
p.m.	post meridiem	evening or afternoon
prn	pro re nata	as needed
p.o.	per os	by mouth or orally
p.r.		by rectum
pulv.	pulvis	powder
q	quaque	every
q.a.d.	quoque alternis die	every other day
q.a.m.	quaque die ante meridiem	everyday before noon
q.h.	quaque hora	every hour
q.h.s.	quaque hora somni	every night at bedtime
q.1h	quaque 1 hora	every 1 hour; (can replace "1" with other numbers)
q.d.	quaque die	everyday
q.i.d.	quater in die	four times a day
q.o.d.		every other day
qqh	quater quaque hora	every four hours

q.s.	quantum sufficiat	a sufficient quantity
R		rectal
rep., rept.	repetatur	repeats
RL, R/L		Ringer's lactate
s	sine	without (usually written with a bar on top of the "s")
s.a.	secundum artum	use your judgement
SC, subc, subq, subcut		subcutaneous
sig		write on label
SL		sublingually, under the tongue
sol	solutio	solution
s.o.s., si op. sit	si opus sit	if there is a need
ss	semis	one half
stat	statim	immediately
supp	suppositorium	suppository
susp		suspension
syr	syrupus	syrup
tab	tabella	tablet
tal., t	talus	such
tbsp		tablespoon
troche	trochiscus	lozenge
tsp		teaspoon
t.i.d.	Ter in die	three times a day
t.d.s.	Ter die sumendum	three times a day
t.i.w.		three times a week
top.		topical
T.P.N.		total parenteral nutrition
tr, tinc., tinct.		tincture
u.d., ut. dict.	ut dictum	as directed
ung.	unguentum	ointment
U.S.P.		United States Pharmacopoeia
vag		vaginally
w		with
w/o		without
X		Times
YO		Years old

REVISION QUESTIONS
Long Answer Type Questions

Q. 1. What is a medical prescription? What are its various parts?

Q. 2. Discuss in brief about various parts of a prescription. Make a prescription showing its various parts.

Q. 3. Enumerate the various steps involved in handling of prescription.

Q. 4. How modern method of prescription is different from old method? What are the advantages and disadvantages of modern method of prescription?

Q. 5. What care is to be taken in writing a prescription?

Q. 6. What are the various sources of error in writing a prescription?

Q. 7. Enumerate the various points which is to be considered in mind for writing a good prescription.

SHORT ANSWER TYPE QUESTIONS

i. The term R_x is an abbreviation of Latin term which means...

ii. The term prescription means ……...……….. a drug can be prepared.

iii. ……...…...……..… is the main part of prescription which contains the name and quantities of prescribed drugs.

iv. Direction for administration of drug to patient comes under ....

v. The color used for labeling "for external use only" is ....

vi. Write the Latin term and meaning of following abbreviation.

		Latin	Meaning
a	a.c.		
b	Alt.h.		
c	Aq		

d	bis		
e	b.i.d.		
f	bol		
g	cc		
h	emuls.		
i	hr		
j	h.s.		
k	liq		
l	nebul		
m	p.c.		
n	p.o.		
o	s.o.s.		
p	t.i.d.		
q	Ung.		

vii. Match the following:

Parts of prescriptio	Significance
1. Date	a. You take
2. Superscription	b. Help in misses of prescription
3. Inscription	c. Direction to patient
4. Signature	d. Name and quantity of medicine

viii. Match the following

Latin term	Meaning
1. Ad	a. Right ear
2. A	b. To make
3. Fiat	c. Mix
4. Mistura	d. Up to
5. Mitte	e. Send

ix. Superscription contains:

i. Symbol R_x
ii. Names and quantities of prescribed ingredients
iii. Instruction to the pharmacist
iv. Direction to the patient

x. Inscription contains:

  i. Symbol R_x

  ii. Direction to the patient

  iii. Names and quantities of prescribed ingredients

  iv. Instruction to the pharmacist.

xi. Modern method of prescribing does not include:

  a. Handover the ready-made preparations to the patients

  b. To advice regarding its mode of administration.

  c. The practice of writing long, complicated prescriptions containing several ingredients.

  d. To advice regarding the quantity of the drug to be taken.

xii. Medicines which are used externally must be labeled **"For external use only"** in:

  a. Red or against a red background

  b. Green or against a green background

  c. Black or against a black background

  d. Yellow or against a yellow background

xiii. Prescription abbreviation used for water is:

  i. aq

  ii. aa

  iii. aa

  iv. ad

xiv. Prescription abbreviation h.s.:

  i. At bedtime

  ii. Hour

  iii. Hypodermic

  iv. None of above

xv. Latin word 'cibos' means:

  i. Food

  ii. With food

  iii. After food

  iv. Before food.

ANSWERS

i. Recipe (you take)
ii. To write before
iii. Inscription
iv. Signatura
v. Red
vii. 1-b, 2-a, 3-d, 4-c
viii. 1-d, 2-a, 3-b, 4-c, 5-e
ix. i
x. iii
xi. c
xii. c
xiii. i
xiv. i
xv. i

7

Incompatibilities in Prescriptions

The prescriptions are generally written for the official and proprietary medicines, which are manufactured by the pharmaceutical industries. The prescriptions are rarely compounded and dispensed in these days in chemist's shop or hospital pharmacy.

"Incompatibility occurs as a result of the mixing of two or more antagonistic substance and an undesirable product is formed which may affect the safety, efficacy and appearance of the pharmaceutical preparation". Incompatibility may occur not only during compounding and dispensing but also at any stage during formulation, manufacturing, packaging or administration of drugs.

Types of Incompatibilities

The incompatibilities are of three types:

1. Physical incompatibility
2. Chemical incompatibility
3. Therapeutic incompatibility

1. PHYSICAL INCOMPATIBILITY

When two or more than two substances are mixed together, a physical change takes place and an unacceptable product is formed. Physical incompatibility is usually due to immiscibility, insolubility, precipitate formation or liquefaction of solid materials. These changes which occur as a result of physical incompatibility are usually visible and can be easily corrected by applying the pharmaceutical skill to obtain a product of uniform dosage, an attractive appearance and having satisfactory therapeutic activity. The physical incompatibilities may be corrected by using any one or more of the following methods:

1. Immiscibility
2. Insolubility
3. Liquefaction

Immiscibility

a. Oils are immiscible with water and hence combination of oily drugs with water produces a product possessing two separate layers.

   Remedy: This problem can be overcome by emulsification or solubilization.

b. Care must be taken when concentrated hydroalcoholic solutions of volatile oils such as spirits and concentrated waters, are used as adjuncts (e.g. as flavoring agents) in aqueous preparations. Large globules of oils may be separated.

   Remedy: To prevent the formation of large globules, the hydroalcoholic solution should either be gradually diluted with the vehicle before admixture with the remaining ingredients or poured into the vehicle with constant stirring.

Insolubility

a. Some insoluble powders such as sulfur and certain corticosteroids (hydrocortisone acetate) and antibiotics are difficult to wet with water.

   Remedy: Wetting agents like saponins for sulfur containing lotions and polysorbates in parenteral suspensions of corticosteroids.

b. When a resinous tincture is added to water the water insoluble resin agglomerate forming indiffusible clots.

   Remedy: This is prevented by slowly adding the undiluted dispersion of protective colloid (tragacanth mucilage), e.g. lobelia and stramonium tincture which should be mixed with tragacanth mucilage and stirred constantly. This will produce a stable preparation.

Liquefaction

When certain low melting point solids are powdered together a liquid or soft mass is produced due to lowering of the melting point of the mixture to below room temperature. Thus, an eutectic mixture is formed. Any two of the following exhibits this type of behavior, camphor, menthol, phenol, thymol and chloral hydrate, also sodium salicylate with phenazone, e.g.

R_x	
Thymol	250 mg
Camphor	2 mg
Menthol	2 mg
Make powder	

Comments: If these ingredients are triturated together, they will form an eutectic mixture.

Method I: All the ingredients are triturated. An eutectic mixture (liquid) will be formed. The liquid is triturated with enough absorbent powder, e.g. light kaolin or light magnesium carbonate, to give a free-flowing powder.

Method II: Each ingredient is triturated separately with small amount of adsorbent or diluent and then these powders are lightly mixed by tumbling action) and packed. The diluent largely prevents contact between the ingredients and adsorbs any liquid that may be produced, e.g.

R_x	
Chloral hydrate	250 mg
Prepare capsules. Supply 10 capsules	
Label: Take the capsules at night time	

Comment: Chloral hydrate is hygroscopic in nature. It will absorb moisture and soften the hard gelatin capsule shells and the shape of the capsule may change physically.

Remedy: An equal quantity of light magnesium oxide should be mixed with chloral hydrate. Other adsorbents those may be used are kaolin, talc, starch, etc.

2. CHEMICAL INCOMPATIBILITY

Chemical incompatibility is due to chemical reactions between the ingredients and a toxic or inactive product may be formed. While dispensing such preperations, precautions should be taken either to prevent the formation of harmful product. Chemical incompatibilities is due to oxidation-reduction, acid base hydrolysis or combination reactions. These reactions leads to precipitation, effervescence, decomposition, color change or by explosion.

Chemical incompatibilities are of two types

1. **Tolerated:** In tolerated incompatibilities, the chemical interaction are minimized by changing the order of mixing or mixing the solutions in dilute forms.

2. **Adjusted:** In adjusted incompatibilities the chemical interaction are prevented by addition or substitution of one of the reacting ingredients of a prescription with another of equal therapeutic value.

The chemical incompatibility may be

i. Intentional: When the prescriber knowingly prescribes the incompatible drugs;

ii. Un-intentional: When the prescriber prescribes the drugs without knowing that there is incompatibility between the prescribed drugs.

EXAMPLES OF CHEMICAL INCOMPATIBILITIES

1. Alkaloidal Incompatibility

i. **Alkaloidal salts with alkaline substances:** Alkaloids are weak bases. They are almost insoluble in water but alkaloidal salts are soluble in water. If these salts are dispensed with alkaline preparations, such as strong solution of ammonium acetate, aromatic spirit of ammonia, solution of ammonia, ammonium bicarbonate, sodium bicarbonate, the free alkaloid may be precipitated.

Example

R_x	
Strychnine hydrochloride solution	6 ml
Ammonium acetate	4 ml
Water up to	120 ml
Make a mixture	

Strychnine hydrochloride is an alkaloidal salt while ammonium acetate is an alkaline substance. When they react together, the strychnine gets precipitated because the quantity of strychnine hydrochloride prescribed in the prescription is much more than its solubility in water. The ammonium acetate contains negligible amount of alcohol which cannot dissolve the strychnine. Hence, it gets precipitated as diffusible precipitate. Hence, follow method A for precipitate yielding combination.

ii. **Alkaloidal salts with salicylates:** When quinine compounds are combined with salicylates, it forms indiffusible precipitates of quinine salicylate.

Example

Quinine hydrochloride	0.12 gm
Sodium salicylate	4.0 gm
Water up to	100 ml

Quinine hydrochloride on reaction with sodium salicylate froms quinine salicylate which gets separated as indiffusible precipitate.

2. Soluble Salicylates Incompatibilities

i. **Soluble salicylates with ferric salt:** Ferric salt reacts with sodium salicylate to liberate indiffusible precipitates of ferric salicylate.

Example

Ferric chloride solution	0.2 ml
Sodium salicylate	0.3 gm
Water up to	9 ml
Make a mixture	

Ferric chloride reacts with sodium salicylate to form ferric salicylate which gets separated as indiffusible precipitate.

3. Chemical Incompatibilities Causing Evolution of Carbon Dioxide Gas

When carbonates or bicarbonates comes in contact of an acid or acidic drug in a mixture, they react together with the evolution of carbon dioxide gas. If the reaction is not allowed to complete before transferring the mixture into a dispensing bottle and corked, there are chances of explosion with bursting of the bottle. To prevent explosion, the reaction must be completed before dispensing the mixture. To speed up the reaction mixed the ingredients in an open vessel and allow the reaction to complete until effervescence ceases.

3. THERAPEUTIC INCOMPATIBILITY

Usually this incompatibility arises when one or more drugs produces response or intensity different from that intended in the patients. It may be due to following below mentioned reasons:

1. Over doses
2. Under doses
3. Contraindicated drugs
4. Drug interactions

1. Over Doses

Excessive single dose: Sometimes a single dose may become overdose depending on the health of the patient, e.g. a normal dose (taking body weight as 70 kg as standard for an adult male) may be overdose for a underweight person, e.g.

R_x	
Atropine sulphate	6 mg
Phenobarbital	360 mg
Make capsules	

Label: One capsule to be taken three times a day before meals.

Remedy: In this prescription the doses of both atropine sulphate and phenobarbital are 12 times the normal doses. The physician intended for 12 capsules to be dispensed but he has mistaken or may be it is an incomplete prescription. Hence, before dispensing the pharmacist should consult the physician again.

Correct prescription

R_x

Atropine sulphate	6 mg
Phenobarbital	360 mg
Make capsules. Supply 12 capsules	

Label: One capsule to be taken three times a day before meals.

Example

R_x

Strychnine sulfate	20 mg
Iron and ammonium citrate	500 mg
Prepare capsules. Supply 12 capsules	

Label: One capsule to be taken three times a day after meals.

Comment: 10 times overdose of strychnine hydrochloride than that of normal. The pharmacist should consult the physician and obtain the permission to change the dose.

Corrected prescription

Strychnine sulphate	2 mg
Iron and ammonium citrate	500 mg
Prepare capsules. Supply 12 capsules	

Label: One capsule to be taken three times a day after meals.

Excessive daily dose: In this case the daily dose of drug is exceeded, e.g.

R_x

Codeine phosphate	15 mg
Ammonium chloride	500 mg
Prepare capsules and supply 24 capsules	

Label: Two capsules to be taken every hour for cough.

Remedy: As per The USP the prescribed dose should be taken after every four hours and not every hour. Hence, the physician should be consulted.

Additive and synergistic combinations: There are certain drugs possessing similar pharmacological activity. If these drugs are combined together, they may produce additive or synergistic action. Hence, the physician should be consulted, e.g.

R_x	
Amphetamine sulphate	20 mg
Ephedrine sulphate	50 mg
Syrup qs	100 ml
Make a mixture	

Label: Take 25 ml every four hours.

Remedy: Both of the drugs have synergistic effect. The formulation will produce overdose effect. Hence, The dose of individual drug should be reduced.

2. Under Dose

In this type of incompatibility, effect of one drug is lessen or antagonized by the presence of another drug. This can be exemplified by combination of following types of drugs:

1. Stimulants like nux vomica, caffeine, etc. with sedatives like barbiturates, paraldehyde, etc.
2. Purgatives like castor oil, liquid paraffin, etc. with antidiarrheal agents like bismuth carbonates.
5. Acidifiers like dilute hydrochloric acid and alkalizers like sodium bicarbonate, magnesium carbonate.

Example

R_x	
Aspirin	300 mg
Probenecid	500 mg
Prepare capsules	

Label: One capsule a day for gout.

Aspirin is an NSAID given to reduce the pain and swelling in case of gout attack. Probenecid blocks the active reabsorption of uric acid from the lumen of nephron, but salicylates (aspirin) blocks this action of probenecid. Hence, both of the drugs are antagonistic to each other, so its combination is therapeutically useless.

3. Contraindicated Drugs

Certain drugs should not be given in particular disease condition, e.g.

i. Corticosteroids are contraindicated in patients with peptic ulcer.

ii. Vasoconstrictors are contraindicated in hypertensive patients

iii. Certain combination of drugs are contraindicate:

R_x	
Sulphadiazine	0.25 gm
Sulphamerazine	0.25 gm
Ammonium chloride	0.50 gm
Prepare capsules	

Label: Take two capsules six hourly for cough.

Comment: In this prescription ammonium chloride is a urinary acidifier and it could cause deposition of sulphonamide crystals in the kidney.

4. Drug Interactions

The effect of one drug is altered by the prior or simultaneous administration of another drug. The drug interactions can usually be corrected by the proper adjustment of dosage if the suspected interaction is detected.

Example

Acetophenetidin	150 mg
Acetyl salicylic acid	200 mg
Caffeine	30 mg
Send ten capsules	

Acetophenetidin and acetyl salicylic acid are analgesics. Acetophenetidin depresses the CNS and this side effect is undesirable. Caffeine is a CNS stimulant to neutralize the side effect of acetophenetidin. The incompatibility is intentional.

Example

R_x

Tetracycline hydrochloride	250 mg
Prepare capsules. Supply 10 capsules	

Label: Take one capsule every six hourly.

Comments: Calcium present in milk inactivates the tetracycline, hence a patient may not get any therapeutic effect if he/she takes the capsule with milk.

Remedy: The pharmacist should advise the patient to take the capsule with water and not with milk. The patient should not take antacid containing calcium salts.

REVISION QUESTIONS
Long Answer Type Questions

Q. 1. What are the various types of incompatibilities in prescription? Discuss in brief.

Q. 2. What is physical incompatibility? How it occurs, give examples?

Q. 3. What is chemical incompatibility? Differentiate between tolerated and adjusted chemical incompatibility.

Q. 4. What is alkaloidal incompatibility? Give some examples.

Q. 5. How chemical incompatibility occur, which involves evolution of carbon dioxide gas?

Q. 6. What is therapeutic incompatibility? Discuss in brief about the various reasons due to which therapeutic incompatibility occurs.

SHORT ANSWER TYPE QUESTIONS

i. Match the following:

Compatibility	Cause
1. Physical	a. Error in writing
2. Chemical	b. Immiscibility
3. Therapeutic	c. Oxidation-reduction

ii. Medicines which are used externally must be labeled **"For external use only"** in:

a. Red or against a red background

b. Green or against a green background

c. Black or against a block background

d. Yellow or against a yellow background

iii. Physical incompatibility may not occur due to:

a. Immiscibility

b. Insolubility

c. Precipitate formation

d. Oxidation

iv. In .... compatibility the chemical interaction are minimized by changing the order of mixing or mixing the solutions in dilute forms:

a. Tolerated

b. Adjusted

c. Intentional

d. Unintentional

ANSWERS

i. 1-b, 2-c, 3-a

ii. a

iii. d

iv. a

8

Extraction and Galenicals

Extraction may be defined as the process in which the animal or plant tissue are treated with specific solvents whereby the medicinally active constituents are dissolved out, cell tissues and most of inactive content remains undissloved. In pharmacy, the solvent used for extraction purposes is known as *menstrum*, and residue left after extracting the desired constituents is known as *marc*.

The products obtained after extractions are impure and intended only for oral and external use. Such preparations include infusions, decoctions, tinctures liquid extracts, semisolid extracts and powder extracts. These types of extracts are known as galenicals after Greek Physician Galen. Previously they were extensively used than at present. They were generally used for extemporaneous dispensing and were required to be freshly prepared.

SOLVENTS USED FOR THE EXTRACTION OF DRUGS

There are a large number of solvents (menstrum) used for extraction of drug but the selection of a suitable solvent capable of extracting the active constitutes depends upon the chemical properties of the active constituents as well as the qualities of solvent. An ideal solvent for the extraction of the drug should be cheap, physically and chemically inert, non-toxic and selective, i.e. it should dissolve only the required constituent with minimum amount of inert materials but these qualities are rarely met. The solvent commonly used for extraction of drugs include water, alcohol and their different dilutions.

A. Water as a Solvent

Water used as a solvent for the extraction of many types of active constituents such a proteins, gums, coloring agents, anthraquinone derivatives, many alkaloidal salts glycosides, sugars and tannins. It can also dissolve enzymes, organic salts and organic acids but cannot dissolve fatty substances such as waxes, fats, fixed oils and alkaloids (as free base).

Advantages

Water as a solvent has the following advantages

i. It is very cheap.

ii. It is non-toxic.

iii. It is non-inflammable.

iv. It can dissolve a wide range of chemical substances.

Disadvantages

i. Water is not selective, as it can dissolve a wide range of substances some of which are not only medicinally inactive but many a times create stability problems.

ii. Water is a good media for the growth of bacteria and molds therefore all preparations made with water must be suitably preserved by adding sufficient quantity of alcohol, chloroform, glycerin or sugar.

iii. Water leads to hydrolysis of many substances.

iv. Liquid extracts prepared with water require more heat for their concentration as compared to extracts prepared with other solvents.

B. Alcohol as a Solvent

Alcohol or ethanol can dissolve a large number of chemical substances such as alkaloids, alkaloidal salts, glycosides, tannins, anthraquinone derivatives, volatile oils and resins but substances like gum, albumin, waxes, fats, most fixed oils, and sucrose are insoluble in alcohol. Generally dilute alcohols (hydroalcoholic solutions) are used for many extractions but in some cases stronger alcohol may be used to prevent extraction of unwanted substances such as gums.

Advantages

Alcohol as solvent has the following advantages

  i. It is miscible with water in all proportions. Various dilutions of alcohol are used for extraction purposes. A mixture of alcohol and alcohol is known as hydroalcoholic solutions.
 ii. It is non-toxic in the quantities present in medicinal substances.
iii. Bacteria and molds cannot grow in solutions containing 20% or more of alcohol.
 iv. Less heat is required for the concentration of extracts prepared in alcohol as compared to that of prepared in water.
  v. It is neutral hence preparations made with it are compatible with other products.
 vi. It is reasonably selective, e.g. in a drug containing a number of chemical substances such as alkaloidal salts, glycosides, albumin and gum, water will dissolve all the substances whereas dilute alcohol will dissolve only the alkaloidal salts and glycosides.

Disadvantages

The main disadvantage of alcohol is that it is costly as compared to water.

The other solvents used for extraction of drugs include ether (anesthetic ether), solvent ether, chloroform, glycerin, light petroleum, acids such as acetic acid and tannic acid and propylene glycol.

EXTRACTION PROCESS

Extraction of crude drugs can be done by various processes depending on the physical nature of the drug and chemical properties of the constituents present in it. Various methods use for extraction of the drugs includes:

1. Infusion
2. Decoction
3. Digestion
4. Maceration
5. Percolation (lixivation)

The processes like infusion, decoction and digestion are now obsolete hence are rarely used with a few exceptions for extraction of drugs. Only the maceration and percolation processes are of particular importance and most pharmacopoeias refer to these processes for extraction of crude drugs.

Infusion

This method is used for those drugs which are soft in nature so that water may penetrate easily to the tissues and the active constituents are water soluble. The simplest form of apparatus consists of a beaker or teapot but special pots known as infusion pots are also available. The drug to be extracted is placed at the bottom of pot, water added and the contents stirred occasionally. Otherwise the drug may be enclosed in a piece of muslin and suspended just below the level of water. The drug is allowed to remain in contact with water for the required time, usually 15 minutes. After the specified time, the liquid is strained and dispensed. The marc is not pressed to avoid expression of colloidal cells into preparation and the final volume of the preparation is not adjusted by adding more of vehicle otherwise dilution of active constituents will take place.

Infusion must be freshly prepared and consumed within 24 hours of its preparation. Examples of infusions are infusion of senna and infusion of quassia. Concentrated infusions are prepared by maceration or percolation process and alcohol is used either as a menstruum or as a preservative. An infusion containing 20–25% alcohol can be stored for sufficient long time. Examples of concentrated infusions are: Concentrated compound infusion of chirata and concentrated compound infusion of gentian.

Decoction

Decoction is the process in which the water soluble and heat stable constituents of hard and woody crude drugs are extracted out. Water is used as menstruum and drug is cut in small pieces is actually boiled with menstruum for the stated time, usually 10 to 15 minutes. After boiling, the liquid is cooled and filtered; more water is passed through marc to produce required volume. Adjustment to final volume is necessary to get a uniform product because different workers will use different types of vessels and different sources of heat resulting in varying losses of water by evaporation. A freshly prepared decoction should only be dispensed and the same must be consumed within 24 hours. At present no decoction is official in BP or IP.

Digestion

This process is a modified form of maceration in which the extraction of drugs is carried out by applying gentle heat to the substances being extracted. This method is applicable only to those drugs where moderately elevated temperature is not objectionable and solvent action of the menstruum is increased by gentle heat.

Maceration

A. **Simple maceration for organized drugs:** Organized drugs are those drugs which have specific cell structure like root, stem, leaves, flowers, etc. In this process the extraction of drugs is carried out by placing solid drug (in suitable state of subdivision, either crushed, cut small or moderately coarse powder. Fine powders are not used because there will be difficulty in subsequent filtration) in contact with whole of the menstruum in a closed vessel for 2 to 7 days with occasional stirring. The liquid is strained and marc pressed, adding the expressed liquid to the stained liquid. The combined liquids are clarified by decantation or filtration. Final volume is not adjusted.

Water or alcohol is sued as menstruum and closed vessel is used to prevent evaporation of menstruum. The drug menstruum ratio is normally 1 : 10. Sufficient time is allowed for menstruum to penetrate plant tissues and for the solubles to diffuse out. Stirring is necessary to disperse concentrated layer of the dissolved constituents around the solid particles. The extracted liquids may contain small particles of insoluble cell contents therefore filtration is necessary to remove these particles but filtration should not be done too soon after extraction, the liquid should be allowed to stand for some time to settle any colloidal material and then filtered otherwise the liquid will again become cloudy due to coagulation of colloidal particles even after filtration. Preparations made by this process include: Oxymel of squill, tincture of squill, tincture of lemon, tincture of orange, etc.

B. Simple maceration for unorganized drugs: Unorganized drugs are those drugs which have no cellular or tissue structure and are obtained from plants as their exudates, e.g. gums, resins, gum resins and oleo gum resin. In this process the extraction of drug is carried out by placing a weighted amount of drug in contact with 4/5th the menstruum in a closed vessel for 2–7 hours with occasional shaking. After the specified period the clear solution is decanted or filtered, marc is not pressed, volume is adjusted by passing more of (remaining 1/5th) menstruum through the marc.

In case of unorganized drugs, the marc left behind after the extraction of active constituents forms a compact mass and does not retain appreciable amount of menstruum therefore pressing the gummy residue is neither practicable nor necessary. The adjustment to volume by washing the gummy residue with more menstruum leads to uniform composition. Preparations made by this process include compound tincture of benzoin, tincture of tolu and tincture of myrrh.

C. Multiple maceration: Repeated maceration may be more effective than single maceration because an appreciable amount of active constituent may be left behind in the first pressing of marc which may be extracted in the next maceration. It is established that the maximum extraction is obtained in multiple maceration when the total quantity of menstruum to be used is divided in such a way that the same quantity of menstruum is present during each maceration. However, allowance must be made for the quantity of menstruum retained by marc at the end of the process. Multiple maceration may be done by double or triple maceration process.

Double maceration: During this process the maceration of drug is carried out twice and the total volume of menstruum is divided into two parts in such a way that the same quantity of menstruum is used for each maceration.

For first maceration the weighed amount of drug is allowed to remain in contact with specified amount of menstruum with occasional shaking for a definite time. After the time is over the liquid is strained and marc pressed, combining the strained and expressed liquid. The second part of menstruum is then added to the marc and allowed to stand for sometime. The clear liquid is strained, marc pressed and liquids obtained from 1st and 2nd maceration combined together, filtered and evaporated together to get a product of required concentration. Concentrated compound infusion of gentian is prepared by double maceration.

The equation for double maceration is

$$\begin{array}{l} \text{Volume of} \\ \text{menstruum to} \\ \text{be used for first} \\ \text{maceration} \end{array} = \frac{\begin{array}{l}\text{Total volume}\\\text{of menstruum}\end{array} - \begin{array}{l}\text{Volume of menstruum}\\\text{retained by the drug}\end{array}}{2}$$

$$+ \begin{array}{l}\text{Volume of mens-}\\\text{truum retained by}\\\text{the drug}\end{array}$$

Triple maceration: Triple maceration process is sometimes used where marc cannot be pressed. As in double maceration, in the case of triple maceration, the menstruum is divided into three parts and maceration is done thrice. The equation for triple maceration is:

$$\begin{array}{l} \text{Volume of} \\ \text{menstruum} \\ \text{required for second} \\ \text{and third maceration} \end{array} = \frac{\begin{array}{l}\text{Total volume}\\\text{of menstruum}\end{array} - \begin{array}{l}\text{Volume of menstruum}\\\text{retained by the drug}\end{array}}{2}$$

$$+ \begin{array}{l}\text{Volume of mens-}\\\text{truum retained by}\\\text{the drug}\end{array}$$

$$\begin{array}{l} \text{Volume of} \\ \text{menstruum} \\ \text{required for second} \\ \text{and third maceration} \end{array} = \frac{\begin{array}{l}\text{Total volume}\\\text{of menstruum}\end{array} - \begin{array}{l}\text{Volume of menstruum}\\\text{used first maceration}\end{array}}{2}$$

In this process a weighed amount of drug is allowed to remain in contact with the calculated amount of menstruum for a specified period of time with occasional shaking, the clear liquid is strained and reserved. Similarly, second and third maceration is carried out by adding calculated quantities of menstruum. The marc is pressed at the end of the third maceration and expressed liquid is mixed with liquids obtained from the 2nd and 3rd maceration. The liquid obtained in the first maceration is quiet concentrated as compared to liquids obtained in 2nd and 3rd maceration hence the later are combined and evaporated before mixing it with the first macerate. Before making up the final volume, alcohol 90% equal to 1/4th of the final volume of liquid to be prepared is added to prevent growth of microorganisms. Liquid extract of senna and concentrated infusion of quassia are prepared by triple maceration process.

Percolation (Lixivation)

Percolation also known as simple percolation is another method of extraction of active constituents from drugs used in preparation of tinctures and liquid extracts. In this process the suitably comminuted drug is moistened with a sufficient quantity of menstruum, which is then packed in a percolator (Fig. 8.1). The drug is allowed remain in contact with menstruum for 24 hours, then more menstruum is added from the top and percolation is started. The required volume is collected, marc pressed and expressed liquid is added to the percolate. The required volume is produced by adding more of menstruum and mixed liquid is clarified by decantation or by filtration. Preparations made by percolation process are: Tincture of belladonna, compound tincture of cardamom, strong tincture of ginger.

The entire percolation process is explained by dividing it into following stages:

Size reduction or comminution of the drug: The drug to be extracted is subjected to suitable degree of size reduction, usually from coarse powder to fine powder; to increase the surface area of the drug, for uniform packing of the percolator, to slow down the movement of the menstruum and to ensure complete exhaustion of the drug.

Imbibition: During imbibition the powdered drug is moistened with a suitable amount of menstruum and allowed to stand for hours in a well-closed container. During this period

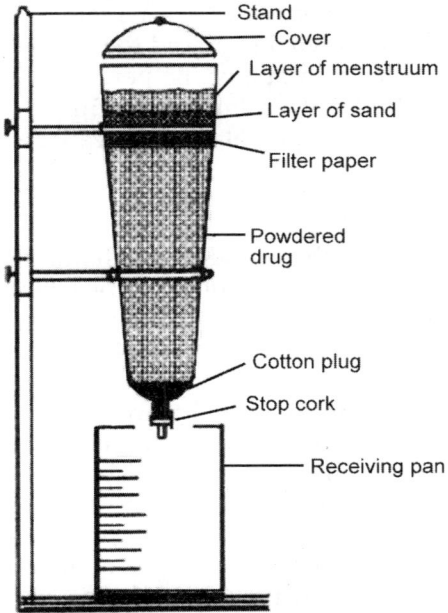

Stand
Cover
Layer of menstruum
Layer of sand
Filter paper
Powdered drug
Cotton plug
Stop cork
Receiving pan

Fig. 8.1: The percolator

the drug swells up and menstruum penetrates the cell walls. After the lapse of time, the moistened drug is passed through a coarse sieve to remove the lumps and to mix the dry powder, if any. This preliminary moistening of the drug is necessary because:

• The dried tissue swells when it come in contact with menstruum but if packed in the dry condition, subsequent swelling will reduce the porosity of the material and choke the percolator.

• The air present in the interstices is removed by menstruum, which will otherwise disturb the packing of the percolator due to which the menstruum will run mainly through channels resulting in inefficient extraction.

• It does not allow the fine particles to be washed out of the percolator during percolation.

Packing: After imbibition the moistened drug is evenly packed into a percolator. A percolator is a conical vessel having a lid at the top and is provided with a false bottom on which filter paper or cotton wool is placed to support the column of the drug and help in escape of the percolate. The base of the percolator is fitted with a tap from which the percolate is collected. Two types of percolator are available:

i. Open percolator

ii. Closed percolator

Open percolator is cheap and easy to handle. It is used when the menstruum is water or dilute alcohol. Closed percolator is used when the menstruum is volatile, e.g. alcohol, ether, etc. IF the percolation is to be carried out at elevated temperatures then steam jacketed percolator may be used. For packing a piece of cotton wool, fibers of flax, hemp, or any other suitable material; previously moistened with menstruum is placed on false bottom of percolator. A small amount of (about 10%) of the moistened drug is introduced into the percolator and is pressed lightly with rod or any other suitable device, to give even compression. Similarly, more of moistened drug is introduced and pressed till whole of drug is packed in the percolator. The packing should not be too tight; it will not allow the menstruum to pass freely which will lead to slow extraction rates. Similarly loose packing will allow menstruum to pass through quickly resulting in incomplete contact with the drug, hence less dissolution of active constituents. Precautions should be taken that the drug should occupy about 2/3rds capacity of the percolator. After suitable packing of the drug into the percolator a piece of filter paper is placed over the top of it on which small quantity of washed sand is placed to prevent disturbance of the packed material.

Maceration: After packing the column, sufficient menstruum is added to saturate the material and top of the percolator is covered with a lid. When the liquid begins to drip from the bottom of the percolator, tap fitted at its bottom is closed. If need arise then more of menstruum is added at the top to maintain a layer of menstruum over the drug. Under no circumstances the column should be allowed to become dry otherwise cracks will appear in the packed column resulting in inefficient percolation. The percolator is then set aside for 24 hours to macerate the drug. This period helps the menstruum to penetrate deep into the tissues and dissolve maximum amounts of active constituents and drug will be extracted with comparatively small amount of menstruum.

Percolation: After 24 hours maceration of the drug, the lower tap is of the percolator is opened and liquid is collected therein is allowed to drip slowly at a controlled speed until 3/4th volume of finished product is obtained. Sufficient menstruum is simultaneously added over the drug because at no time packed material should be allowed to become dry. To avoid adding the menstruum time and again, a bottle full of menstruum carrying a delivery tube to the percolator may be fitted in the inverted position which will supply the menstruum continuously over the top of the percolator. After collecting 3/4th volume, the percolate is tested for complete exhaustion of drug by various test, marc is then pressed and expressed liquid is added to the already collected percolate which should be 80–90% of the final volume. More of menstruum is added to produce the required volume. The liquid is then allowed to stand to settle the suspended particles, decanted or clarified by filtration.

Test to check complete exhaustion of the drug

- Take a few ml of the last percolate and evaporate to dryness, if no residue remains this shows that the drug is completely exhaustion.
- Measure the specific gravity of last of percolate if it is equal to specific gravity of the menstruum, it shows exhaustion of the drug.
- Specific test may be performed on the percolate for the drugs containing alkaloids, glycosides, tannins, resins or bitter constituents.

Reserved Percolation

It is a percolation process in which first portion (about 3/4ths of the final product) of the percolate which contains the maximum amount of active constituents is reserved and subsequent percolation is completed as usual until drug is exhausted but the last part, about 1/4th of the final volume is collected separately. The second dilute part is then evaporated to get a syrupy consistency which is then mixed with the reserved portion of percolate and final volume is adjusted by adding more of menstruum.

Reserved percolation process is used in preparation of liquid extracts as they are more concentrated preparations as compared to tinctures prepared by simple percolation process. Generally alcohol is used as menstruum for reserved percolation process and first portion which the bulk of dissolved active constituents is reserved and only the last portion which is dilute is subjected to evaporation, the concentrated product of which is mixed with the reserved part. Liquid extract of liquorice is prepared by this process.

Advantages

* The reserved part of percolate which contains the maximum amount of dissolved principle is not subjected to heat treatment for evaporation; only dilute portion of percolate is evaporated.
* This process is economical as a whole of the percolate is not evaporated.

Continuous Hot Percolation Process or Soxhlet Extraction

Continuous hot percolation process is used for those drugs where penetration of the menstruum into the cellular tissues is very slow and the solute is not readily soluble into the solvent and the quantity of menstruum is very less. In such cases Soxhlet extractor is used where small volume of hot menstruum is passed over the drug time and again to dissolve out the active constituents until drug is exhausted. This process is known as soxhlation.

The soxhlet apparatus required for continuous hot percolation is made of very high grade glass and consist of three parts

a. A flask in which the menstruum is boiled
b. An extraction chamber in which drug is filled, is fitted with a side tube and a siphon
c. A condenser.

The dried sample weighed into porous cellulose thimble. The thimble is placed in an extraction chamber, which is suspended above a flask containing the solvent and below a condenser. The flask is heated and the solvent evaporates and moves up into the condenser, where it is converted into a liquid that trickles into the extraction chamber containing the sample-extracting the active constituents. The extraction chamber is designed so that when the solvent surrounding the sample exceeds a certain level it overflows and trickles back down into the boiling flask—cycle is repeated. At the end of the extraction process, lasting a few hours, the flask containing the solvent and extract is removed. The solvent in the flask is then evaporated and the mass of the remaining extract is measured. In some device a funnel allows to recover the solvent at the end of the extraction after closing a stopcock between the funnel and the extraction chamber (Fig. 8.2).

Working

The drug to be extracted, in suitably comminuted is usually packed in a 'thimble' made of filter paper which is then placed into the wider part of the extractor. 'Thimble' is used to prevent

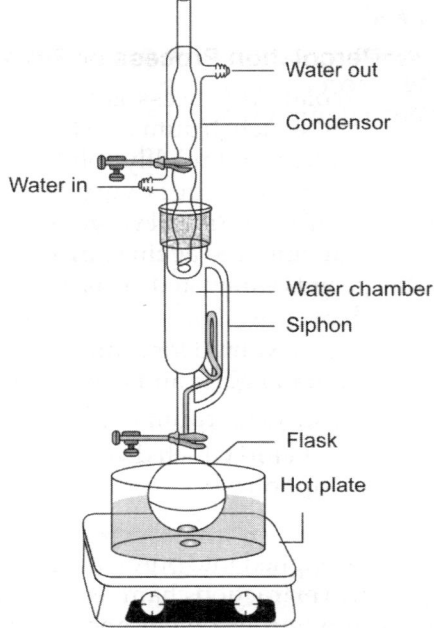

Fig. 8.2: Soxhlet apparatus

choking of the lower part of the extractor by drug particles. Menstruum is placed in the flask and boiled, the vapors are allowed to pass through the side tube to the condenser where they are condensed and fall onto the packed drug, through which it percolates and extract out the active constituents. As the volume of menstruum in the extractor increases, level of the liquid in the siphon also increases till it reaches a maximum point where it is siphoned out into the flask. The alternate filling and emptying of the body of the extractor goes on continuously till the drug is exhausted. Thus, the same quantity of menstruum is made to percolate repeatedly, about 14 to 15 times through the drug and the active constituents are collected in flask. This process is not suitable for drugs containing thermolabile active constituents.

FACTORS AFFECTING EXTRACTION PROCESS

The final choice of the process to be used for the extraction of a drug will depend on a number of factors which are as follows:

1. **Character of drug:** The knowledge of pharmacognosy of the drug is essential to select the right method of extraction process. The maceration process is used when the drug is soft, unorganized, unpowderable and to avoid powdering of it. The percolation process is used when the drug is hard and tough.

2. **Therapeutic value of the drug:** When the drug has considerable therapeutic value, the maximum extraction is required, so the percolation process is used, e.g. (belladonna). In case the drug has a little therapeutic value. The efficiency of extraction is unimportant and maceration process can be used to extract the drug.

3. **Cost of drug:** The costly drugs are extracted by using the percolation process, whereas cheap drugs are extracted by maceration process.

4. **Stability of drug:** Continuous hot extraction process should be avoided when the constituents of the drug are thermolabile in nature. In that case maceration or percolation process may be used to extract the active constituents of the drug.

5. **Solvent:** If water is used to a solvent the maceration process would be recommended. The percolation process should be preferred if non-aqueous solvents are used for extraction. If the desired active constituents of drug demand a solvent other than. A pure boiling solvent or an azeotrope, continuous hot extraction process should be avoided and reserve percolation process may be used.

6. **Concentration of product:** The dilute products such as tinctures can be made by using maceration or percolation process, depending on the other factors, for semi-concentrated preparations, such as concentrated infusions, double of triple maceration process can be used. The liquid extracts or dry extracts which are concentrated preparation are prepared by using percolation process (Tables 8.1 to 8.4).

Table 8.1: Comparison of maceration process for organized drugs and unorganized drugs

Organized drugs	Unorganized drugs
1. Drug along with the whole of the menstruum is used in maceration process	1. Drug along with 4/5ths of the menstruum is used in maceration process
2. The period of maceration is 7 days	2. The period of maceration is 2–7 days
3. Strain off the liquid and press the marc	3. Decant the liquid. Marc is nor pressed
4. Mix the pressed liquid with the macerate and clarify by subsidence or filtration. Filtrate is not adjusted to volume	4. Filter the liquid and pass the remaining 1/5th of menstruum through filter to make up the final volume
5. Examples of tinctures made by this process are: a. Tincture of orange b. Tincture of lemon c. Tincture of capsicum	5. Examples of tinctures made by this process are: a. Compound tincture of benzoin b. Tincture of tolu c. Tincture of myrrh

Table. 8.2: Comparison between maceration process and infusion process

Maceration	Infusion process
1. Menstruum used is usually alcohol, but it may be aqueous	1. Cold or boiling water is used as menstruum

Contd.

Table. 8.2: Comparison between maceration process and infusion process *(Contd.)*

Maceration	Infusion process
2. Drug is made in contact with menstruum for 2–7 days	2. Drug is made in contact with menstruum for 15 minutes
3. The process is conducted at room temperature	3. The process may or may not be conducted at room temperature
4. Marc is pressed after maceration except is modified maceration process	4. Marc is not pressed
5. Volume is not made up in simple maceration but adjustment to volume is done in modified maceration process	5. Volume is not made in infusion process

Table 8.3: Comparison between infusion and decoction

Infusion	Decoction
1. Cold or boiling water is used as menstruum	1. Drug is boiled in water
2. Drug having soft tissue is used	2. Drug of a hard tissue is used
3. Drug constituents may be volatile	3. Drug constituents should be nonvolatile
4. Final volume is not adjusted	4. Adjustment to volume is done
5. When boiling water is used as menstruum, precautions are taken to prevent the escape of heat by covering the vessel with a cloth	5. No such precaution is required because the final volume

Table 8.4: Comparison between double maceration and triple maceration

Double maceration	Triple maceration
1. Menstruum is divided into two parts	1. Menstruum is divided into three parts
2. The drugs is macerated for 48 hours in first maceration followed by second maceration.	2. The drug is macerated thrice having each maceration of one hour duration
3. Strain the liquid after each maceration and press the marc.	3. Strain the liquid after each maceration and press the marc after the last laceration

Contd.

Table 8.4: Comparison between double maceration and triple maceration (Contd.)

Infusion	Decoction
4. The pressed liquid after is mixed with the strained liquids of both macerations and then the volume is adjusted after adding more of menstruum	4. Combine the strained liquid obtained from the second and the third maceration evaporate it to a specified extent. Mix it with strained liquid obtained after first maceration. Add alcohol 90% equal to 14th of the volume of the finished product
5. Alcohol 25% is used as menstruum	5. Water is used as meanstruum but alcohol 90% is added at the end equal to 1/4th of the volume of the finished product

KEY POINTS

Maceration (for fluid extract)

- Whole or coarsely powdered plant-drug is kept in contact with the solvent in a stoppered container for a defined period with frequent agitation until soluble matter is dissolved
- The mixture is strained, the marc pressed and the combined liquid filtered.

Percolation (for tinctures and fluid extracts)

- Percolator (a narrow, cone-shaped vessel open at both ends) is used
- The powdered drug is moistened with an appropriate amount of the specified menstruum and allowed to stand for 4 h in
- Well-closed container
- The moistened mass loosely packed in percolator and covered
- Additional menstruum added to give shallow layer above the mass
- Allowed to macerate for 24 hours
- Outlet of the percolator opened and liquid allowed to drip slowly
- Additional menstruum being added as required, until the percolate measures about three quarter of the required volume
- Marc is pressed, liquid added to the percolate and sufficient menstruum added to the required volume and filtered.

Infusion

- Infusion is dilute solution of the readily soluble constituents of the crude drug
- Fresh infusion is prepared by macerating the drug for a short period of time with cold or hot (boiling) water.

Digestion

- It is like maceration but gentle heat is used during the process of extraction
- It is employed when moderately elevated temperature is not objectionable as the solvent efficiency is increased.

Decoction

- Powdered drug is boiled in specified volume of water for defined time, cooled and strained or filtered
- Suitable for extracting water-soluble, heat stable constituents
- Most widely used process for Ayurved drugs and is called "Quath"
- Ratio of drug to water 1 : 4 or 1 : 16 which is brought down to ¼ of its original volume by boiling.

HOT CONTINUOUS EXTRACTION (SOXHLET)

Process

- Finely powdered crude drug held in porous bag (thimble) placed in chamber.
- Extracting solvent in flask heated
- Vapours condensed in condenser
- Condensed solvent drips into the thimble containing drug, extracting it by contact
- As the level of the liquid in chamber rises to the top of the siphon tube, the liquid contents of siphon into flask
- The process is continued until a drop of solvent from the siphon tube, when evaporated, does not leave a residue.

Advantages

- Large amount of drug can be extracted with much smaller quantity of solvent

- Tremendous economy in terms of time, energy and ultimately financial inputs
- Small scale used a batch-process
- Becomes more economical when converted into continuous extraction procedure on large scale.

PRACTICE QUESTIONS
Very Short Answer Type Questions

1. What are the various processes used in the extraction of crude drugs?

2. What does the term "extraction" mean?

3. Define the term "menstruum", and "marc".

4. Prepare a list of the different types of menstruum used in the extraction of crude drugs.

5. Why is stirring of the drug required during infusion and maceration processes?

6. Why is coarse powder of drug used in the infusion process?

7. Why should fresh infusion be used in 12 hours after its preparation?

8. Why the marc is pressed in various extraction processes?

9. Why is the marc not pressed in the maceration process for unorganized drugs?

10. Which type of drugs cannot be extracted by soxhlation process?

11. Why boiling water is commonly used a solvent in infusion process.

Short Answer Type Questions

12. Enlist the advantages and disadvantages of water as a solvent.

13. Give the advantages and disadvantages of alcohol as a solvent.

14. Describe different type of maceration process.

15. Define the term "percolation".

16. Why is a short period of maceration required before the actual percolation process?

17. Write the advantages of a conical percolator.

18. What are the advantages of a cylindrical percolator?

19. Why is imbibition done before packing of the drug into the percolator?

20. Why is maceration done in a covered vessel?

21. Describe various percolation processes for extraction of drug.

22. What are the various steps in packing of a drug in a percolator?

23. Mention the various limitations of continuous hot percolation process.

Long Answer Type Questions

24. Describe in detail the simple maceration process for extraction of crude drugs. Explain as to how it differs from the modified maceration process.

25. Describe the process of simple percolation used in the preparation of tinctures.

26. What is reserve percolation? How is it carried out?

27. What is multiple maceration? What are its merits and demerits?

28. Describe the process of infusion. Discuss the different types of infusions.

29. Differentiate between the following:
    a. Infusion and decoction
    b. Infusion and maceration
    c. Double maceration and triple maceration
    d. Simple maceration and multiple maceration
    e. Maceration process for organized drugs and unorganized

30. Write short notes on:
    a. Infusion   b. Decoction
    c. Maceration   d. Percolation
    e. Reserve percolation process   f. Soxhlation
    g. Multiple maceration process   h. Digestion

Objective Type Questions

31. Alcohol in the conc. of .... is used as .... in multiple maceration process.

32. One volume of conc. infusion when diluted with .... volume of water resembles the corresponding fresh infusion in ....

33. The process of extraction in which the drug is kept in contact with menstruum for 15 minutes is called ....

34. Simple maceration is done in a covered vessel for .... days to prevent .... of menstruum which is mostly .... in nature.

35. In double maceration process, the whole of the drug is macerated for .... with a part of menstruum and then it is macerated again for .... with the remaining menstruum.

36. In soxhlation process .... solvent or .... mixtures are used.

37. When a drug is extracted by heating at a particular pressure the process is called ....

38. Match the items of column I with appropriate terms in column II.

Column I	Column II
A. Concentrated infusion	I Unsuitable for drugs having
B. Multiple maceration process	II For preparation of tinctures from organized drugs
C. Soxhlation process	III The drug is boiled with solvent
D. Decoction	IV Prepared by double or triple maceration
E. Simple maceration process	V Used for preparation of conc. preparation
F. Compound tincture of benzoin	VI Prepared by simple maceration
G. Tincture of orange	VII Conc. of alcohol is 20.25%
H. Double maceration	VIII Prepared by maceration process for unorganized drug

31. 20–25% menstruum.

32. Seven, potency.

33. Infusion.

34. Seven, evaporation, volatile.

35. 48 hours, 24 hours.

36. Pure, constant boiling mixtures.

37. Digestion.

38. A (iv), B (v), C (i), D (iii), E (ii), F (viii), G (vi), H (vii).

9

Mixing

Mixing is the most widely used operation in which two or more than two substances are combined together. Perfect mixing is that in which each particles of one material lies as nearly as possible to a particles of the other material. Mixing may be defined as the process in which two or more than two components in a separate or roughly mixed condition are treated in such a way so that each particle of any one ingredient lies as nearly as possible to the adjacent particles of other ingredients or components. This process may involve the mixing of gases, liquids or solids in any possible combination and in any possible ratio of two or more components.

Objectives of Mixing

a. To ensure uniformity of composition so that smallest quantity of sample taken from any corner of the bulk represents overall composition of the mixture. To ensure that there is uniformity of composition between the mixed ingredients which may be determined by taking samples from the bulk material and analyzing them, which should represent overall composition of the mixture.

b. To facility dispersion of two immiscible liquids to form emulsion and dispersion of solid in liquid forming suspension or paste. Mixing is required to ensure stability and uniformity.

c. Mixing will usually encourage and control chemical reaction and ensure uniform product.

d. To initiate or to enhance the physical or chemical reactions, e.g. diffusion, dissolution, etc.

203

Types of products obtained after mixing: Following type of products are obtained after mixing:

a. When two or more than two miscible liquids are mixed together, this results into a solution known as *true solution*.

b. When two immiscible liquids are mixed in the presence of an emulsifying agent, an *emulsion* is produced.

c. When a solid is dissolved in a liquid, a *solution* is obtained

d. When an insoluble solid is mixed with a liquid, a *suspension* is obtained.

e. When a solid or liquid is mixed with a semisolid base, an *ointment or a suppository* is produced.

f. When two or more than two solid substances are mixed together, a *powder* is obtained.

Factors Affecting mixing

Particle and powder characteristics influence the mixing process. Aggregation inhibits proper mixing. A single factor is not responsible for proper mixing. However, flow properties of the components are the most important consideration which is again influenced by a number of factors.

1. **Particles shape and surface:** Rough surface of one of the components does not induce satisfactory mixing. This can be due to the entry of active substance into the pores of the other ingredients. The ideal particles are spherical in shape for the purpose of uniform mixing. The irregular shapes can become inter locked and there are less chances of separation of particles once these are mixed together

2. **Adding a substance:** Which will be adsorbed on its surface, can decrease aggregation. Example is the addition of aerosil (colloidal silicon dioxide) to zinc oxide. Thus, a strongly aggregation zinc oxide becomes a fine dusting powder, which can be mixed easily.

3. **Density of the particles:** It is of minor importance. Remixing is accelerated when the density of the smaller particles is higher or when the mixing process is stopped abruptly. This is due to the fact that dense material always moves downward and settles at the bottom.

4. **Particle size:** It is easy to mix two powders having approximately the same particle size. The variation of particle size can lead to separation, because the small particles move downward through the spaces between the bigger particles. As the particles increase, flow properties also increase due to the influence of gravitational force on the size. Beyond a particular point, flows property decrease. The powders with a mean particles size of less than 100 μm are free flowing, which facilities mixing.

5. **Particles charge:** Some particles exert attractive forces due to electrostatic charges on them. This can lead to separation or segregation.

6. **Proportion of materials:** The best results can be obtained if two powders are mixed in equal proportion by weight and by volume. If there is a large difference in the proportion of two powders, mixing is always done in the ascending order of their weights.

Types of Mixtures

There are three types of mixtures:

i. Positive mixtures
ii. Negative mixtures
iii. Neutral mixtures.

i. **Positive mixtures:** When two or more than two miscible liquids are mixed or soluble solid is dissolved in water, the mixtures are called positive mixtures. These mixtures do not present any problem in mixing. The mixture formed in this way is irreversible.

ii. **Negative mixtures:** When two immiscible liquids are mixed or insoluble solids are mixed with water it forms negative mixtures. For preparing such types of mixtures a higher degree of mixing of materials is required. The mixture formed in this way is reversible mixture.

iii. **Neutral mixtures:** These mixtures are inert in their behavior. The substances do not have the tendency to mix with each other immediately, but once mixed they do not separate after mixing.

Classification of Mixer

Mixers classified on the basis of physical state of material to be mixed, and rotational devices (Table 9.1 and Flow chart 9.1):
1. Liquid mixers
2. Solid mixers (powder mixers)
3. Semi-solid mixers.

Table 9.1: Classification of mixing equipment

S. No.	Type of mixing	Name of the mixer	Uses
1.	Liquid-liquid mixing	Shaker mixers, propeller mixers, paddle mixers, turbine mixers, sonic and ultrasonic devices like rapisonic homogenizer	Used in the preparation of emulsions, antacid suspensions, mixtures such as anti-diarrheal bismuth-kaolin mixtures, etc. Rapisonic homogenizer is used for the mixing of immiscible liquids, i.e. like emulsions
2.	Solid-solid mixing	Agitator mixers, tumbling mixers, double-cone mixers, V-blenders	Used for the mixing of dry powders
3.	Semi-solid mixing	Agitator mixers like sigma mixers and planetary mixers, shear mixers like colloidal mills and triple roller mills	Used for wet granulation process in the manufacture of tablets, in the production of ointments. Sigma mixers can also be used for solid-solid mixing

Flow chart 9.1: Classification of mixing equipment

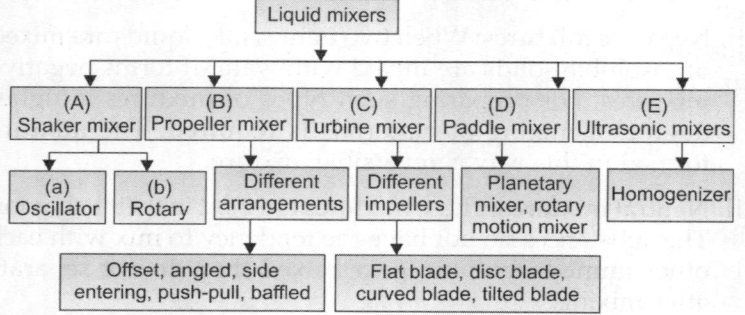

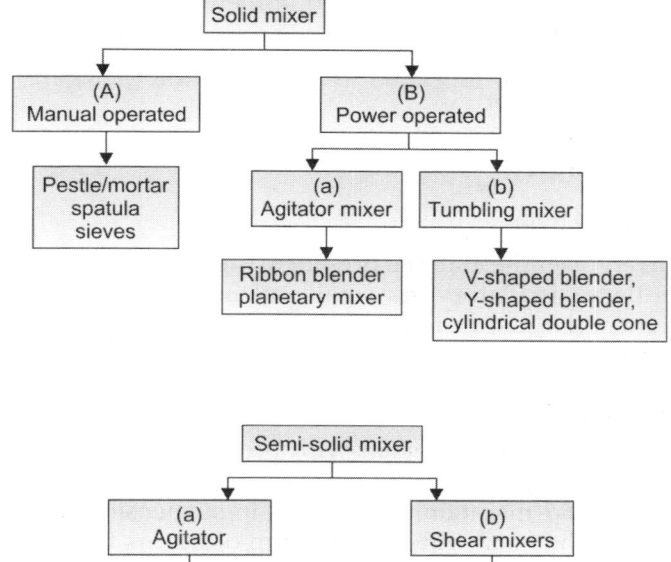

LIQUID-LIQUID MIXING

Mixing of liquids is done to prepare true solution or emulsions. Mixing is required to dissolve one miscible liquid into another miscible liquid to form true solution. For making emulsion, the mixing of two immiscible liquids are done by using shear force.

Equipment Used for Mixing of Liquids

In the laboratory the emulsion is prepared by using pestle and mortar and afterward it is passed through a homogenizer to get fine emulsion. Equipment such as shaker mixers, propeller mixers, turbine mixers and paddle mixers are used for liquid mixing. These equipment contain a flat bottomed, unbaffled or baffled cylindrical vessel with tank diameter to liquid ratio usually as 1 : 1. The vessel is generally made of stainless steel for pharmaceutical operations. Impellers are mixing devices that include paddles, turbines and vaned discs.

On large scale, the following equipment are used for mixing the liquids:

1. Shaker mixer
2. Propeller mixer
3. Turbine mixer
4. Paddle mixer.

1. Shaker Mixer

In shaker mixer the material present in the containers is agitated either by an oscillatory (for small scale mixing) or by a rotary movement (large scale mixing). Shaker mixers have limited use in industry.

2. Propeller Mixer

It consists of a rotating shaft with propeller blades attached, used for mixing relatively low viscosity dispersions (thicker solutions) and maintaining contents in suspension. Propeller mixers are the most widely used form of mixers for liquids of low viscosity. It rotates at a very high speed, i.e. up to 8000 rpm due to which mixing is done in a short time. They are much smaller in diameter than paddle and turbine mixers. During mixing of liquids, air gets entrapped in liquids or there is formation of vortex. This can be avoided by making the following changes in the position of the propeller shaft (Fig. 9.1).

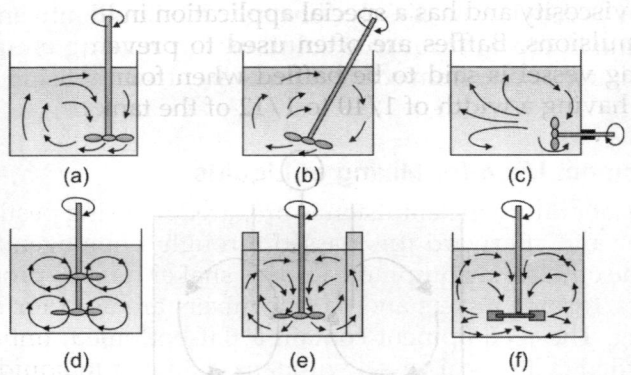

Fig. 9.1: Liquid-liquid mixing: (a) Offset from the center; (b) Mounted at angle; (c) Side of the vessel; (d) Using push-pull propeller; (e) Use of baffles; (f) Turbine

a. Offset from the center
b. Mounted at angle
c. Enter the side of the vessel
d. Using push-pull propeller
e. By the use of baffles
f. Turbine

Uses of propeller mixers: Propellers are used when high mixing capacity is needed. These are effective in handling liquids having a viscosity of about 2.0 Pascal. second.

Disadvantage: Propellers are not effective with liquids of viscosity greater than 5 Pascals second for example, glycerin and castor oil. The propeller mixers are not suitable for the preparation of emulsion.

3. Turbine Mixers

It consists of a vessel and a circular disc impeller. A number of short, straight or curved blades are attached to it. The turbine impeller is usually rotated at somewhat lower speed than the propeller. The turbine mixer is used for mixing of more viscous liquids, e.g. syrups, liquid paraffin, glycerin, etc. (Fig. 9.2). These mixers differ from propellers in that they are rotated at a lower speed than propellers and the ratio of the impeller and container diameter is also low. The former produces greater shear forces than propellers therefore they are used for mixing liquids of high viscosity and has a special application in the preparation of emulsions. Baffles are often used to prevent vortexes. A mixing vessel is said to be baffled when four vertical strips, each having a width of 1/10 to 1/12 of the tank diameter, are

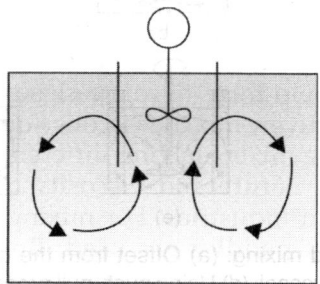

Fig. 9.2: Turbine mixer in a baffled tank

attached to the internal surface of the cylindrical container perpendicularly at 90 degrees position. If solids are present, the baffles are fixed with a gap of about 1 inch between the baffle and the vessel wall.

Turbine mixers are highly efficient. They can bring rapid blending of low viscosity materials of large volumes, produce intense dispersion type agitation in large volumes and can bring about efficient dispersion in multi-liquid phase systems. They can handle slurries containing up to a maximum viscosity of 7,00,000 cps. They can also handle fibrous slurries containing about 5% of the dispersion volume.

In general, it can be said that propeller in a baffled tank is principally a mixing device to handle relatively low volumes of low viscosity liquids while turbine is a very efficient shearing device that can handle very large volumes of liquids of relatively high viscosity. The high shearing at the tip of the blades of a turbine rotating in a baffled vessel is produced due to the radial flow pattern where in the periphery of the blades move in a circular fashion while the liquid is thrown out horizontally towards the surface of the vessel.

Uses of turbine mixers: Turbines are effective for high viscous solutions with a wide range of viscosities up to 700 Pascal. seconds.

Advantage: Turbines give greater shearing forces than propellers and thus they are more suitable for preparation of emulsions.

4. Paddle Mixer

In a paddle mixer, the flat blades are attached to a vertical shaft which rotates at a low speed of 100 rpm. The blades have a large surface area in relation to the container in which they are employed which help them to rotate close to the walls of the container and effectively mix the viscous liquids or semi-solids. A variety of paddle mixers having different shapes and sizes, depending on the nature and viscosity of the product are available for use in industries. For mixing the low viscosity liquids simple flat paddles are used. But for mixing high viscosity liquids, the big paddles, often shaped to fit closely to the surface of the vessel are used. The paddles of different sizes are used in the pharmaceutical industry according to the character and viscosity of the product.

Uses

Paddle mixer are used in the manufacture of antacid suspensions, anti-diarrheal mixtures such as bismuth-kaolin mixture.

Advantage: Since mixers with paddle-impellers have low speed, vortex formation is not possible with such mixers.

Disadvantage: Mixing of the suspensions is poor, thus, baffled tanks are required.

SOLID-SOLID MIXING

The mixing of powders is one of the common pharmaceutical operations and is used in the preparation of many types of formulations, such as, tablets, capsules and compound powders. The solid mixing takes place by a combination of one or more mechanism given below:

1. **Convective mixing:** There is bulk movement of groups of particles from one part of powder bed to another. It occurs by an inversion of the powder bed by means of blades or paddles.

2. **Shear mixing:** When shear forces occur it reduces the scale of segregation by thinning of dissimilar layers of a solid material.

3. **Diffusion mixing:** It occurs when random motion of particles within a powder bed causes them to change position relative to one another. It is produced by any form of agitation of powder.

There are various physical properties, which affect the perfect mixing of powders. These are discussed hereunder:

1. **Particle size:** It is easy to mix two powders having approximate the same particle sizes. If there is variation of particle size it can lead to separation of particles whereby the small particles move downward through the spaces between the bigger particles.

2. **Particle shape:** The ideal particle shape is spherical for the purpose of uniform mixing. The irregular shapes can

become interlocked and there are less chances of separation of particles once these are mixed together.

3. **Particle attraction:** Some particles develop charges due to these charges they exert attractive forces which leads to separation and aggregation of particles leading to variation in particles size.

4. **Material density:** It is difficult to mix two powders having different density. This is due to the fact that dense material always moves downward and settles down at the bottom. Hence, in order to have uniform mixing particle density is to be taken in consideration.

5. **Quantity of materials:** The best results can be achieved if two powders are mixed in equal proportions by weight or by volume. In case there is a large difference in the proportion of two powders to be mixed the mixing of powders is always dome in the ascending order of their weights.

Equipment Used for Mixing of Powders

In the laboratory, the mixing of powders is done by using pestle and mortar or with the help of a drug spatula. The method is commonly known as 'trituration'. On large scale, the following equipment are used for mixing of powders:

1. Dry mixer
2. Vertical screw mixer
3. Agitator mixer
4. Tumble mixer
5. Double cone mixer
6. V-Blender.

1. Dry Mixer

It consists of a semi-cylindrical trough, usually covered and provided with two or more ribbon spirals. One spiral is right-handed and the other left-handed (Fig. 9.3). Ribbon cross-section and number of spirals on the ribbon are varied depending upon the type of material like low density, finely divided materials to fibrous or sticky materials. It may be center discharge or end discharge. Another variation is the mounting of cutting blades on the central shaft. A broad ribbon lifts and conveys the materials while a narrow one will cut through the materials while conveying. Ribbon blenders are often used on the large scale and may be adapted for continuous mixing (Fig. 9.4).

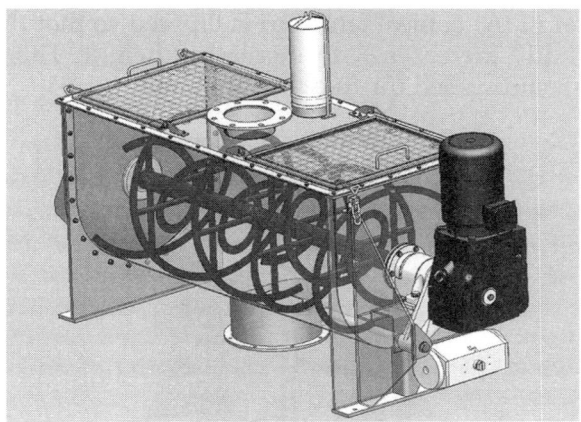

Fig. 9.3: Dry mixer

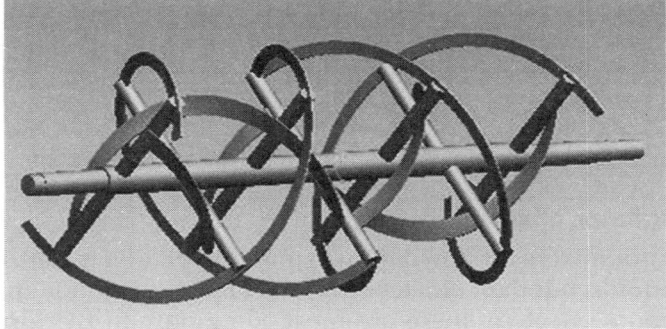

Fig. 9.4: Blades of dry mixer in the form of ribbon

The paddle mixer has a stationary outer vessel and the powders are agitated by paddles rotating within. The equipment is suitable to heating, by jacketing the vessel, and also permits a kneading effect by the use of appropriately shaped paddles or beaters. In the bowl mixer the paddle is mounted vertically and in the trough mixer (e.g. dry mixer) a number of vanes are mounted horizontally.

2. Vertical Screw Mixer

In these types of mixers, the screw rotates about its own axis while orbiting around the center axis of the conical tank (Fig. 9.5). In another variation, the screw does not orbit but remains in the center of the conical tank and is tapered so that the swept area steadily increases with increasing height. This type of mixer is mainly used for free-flowing solids.

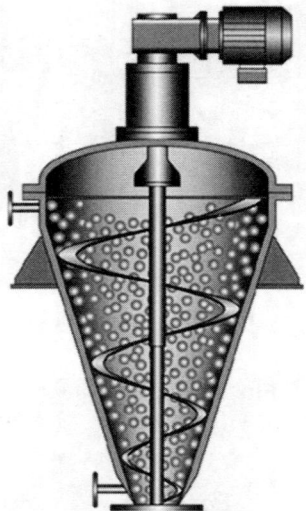

Fig. 9.5: Vertical screw mixer

3. Agitator Mixer

Agitator mixers for powders are similar to paddle mixers used for liquids, but their efficiency is low. Planetary motion mixers are more effective, these are most commonly in the form of trough in which an arm rotates and transmits shearing action to the particles. General mixing requires an end-to-end movement which can be obtained by fitting helical blades to the agitator. In these mixers shear forces are not high, so that aggregates may remain unbroken and the movement may encourage segregation due to density or size differences. This type of mixer is most suitable for blending free-flowing materials, with components that are of uniform size and density (Fig. 9.6).

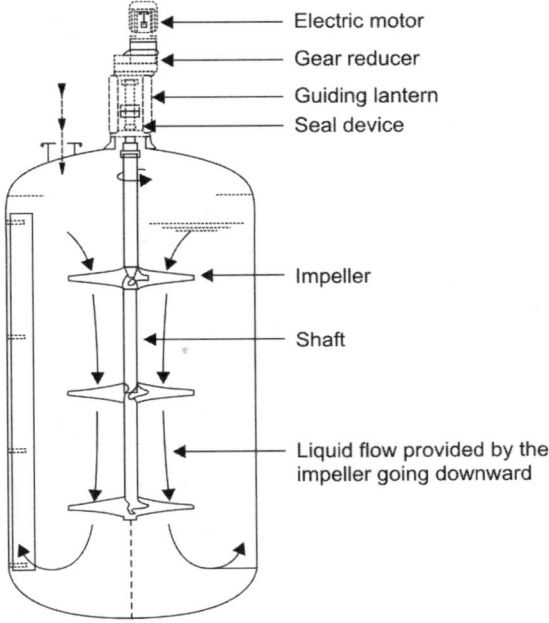

- Electric motor
- Gear reducer
- Guiding lantern
- Seal device
- Impeller
- Shaft
- Liquid flow provided by the impeller going downward

Fig. 9.6: Agitator mixer

4. Tumbler Mixer

In tumbling mixers, rotation of the vessel imparts movement to the materials by tilting the powder until the angle of the surface exceeds the angle of repose when the surface layers of the particles go into a slide. Simple forms use a cylindrical vessel rotating on its horizontal axis, but shear forces are low and end-to-end movement is slight. This may be overcome by including flights (a form of baffles), or the shape of the vessel may be altered to avoid symmetry. A number of different designs are used, such as a cylinder rotating about its mid-point on an axis at right angles to the longitudinal axis, a cube rotating about a diagonal and double-cone, V-shape, Y-shape or diamond shaped vessels, together with baffles where appropriate. These shapes give effective three-dimensional movement and shearing takes place as the charge flows. In addition, the particles hit against the wall and are deflected, causing considerable velocity and acceleration gradients. The repeated reversal of the direction of flow makes the tumbling mixer preferable where differences in density for particle size occur.

5. Double-Cone Mixer

A variety of equipment is available in which the container rotates. This may consist of horizontal rotating cylindrical drum with deep or cupped flights on the inside. When drum is rotated slowly, the powders cascade over one another. With a plain drum, the mixing is not efficient when the proportions and characteristics of the powders vary widely. A double-cone mixer consists of a vessel with two cones base to base, with or without a cylindrical section in between as shown in Figs 9.7a and b. It is so mounted that it can be rotated about an axis at right angles to the line joining the points of the cones. Tumblers of this type are available plain or with an agglomerate-breaking device or with a spray nozzle or with both of these devices. Mechanism of mixing in a double cone mixer is illustrated in Fig. 9.8.

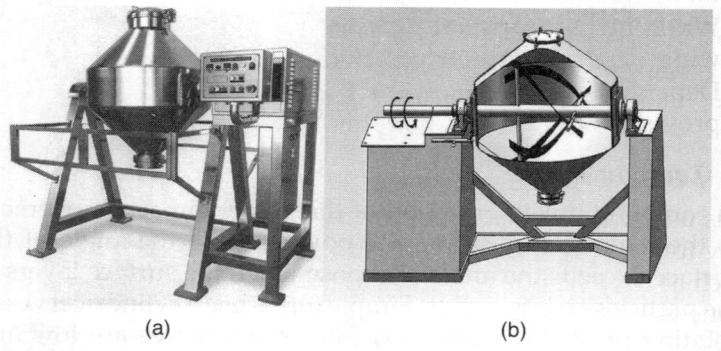

(a)   (b)

Figs 9.7a and b: (a) Double-cone mixer, (b) Internal view of double-cone mixer

Double-cone mixer is an efficient mixer for mixing dry powder and granulates homogeneously. All the contact parts are made up of stainless steel. Two-thirds of the volume of the cone blender is filled to ensure proper mixing.

Features

- The mixing barrel and blades are made of stainless steel, always keeping clean and away from dirt.

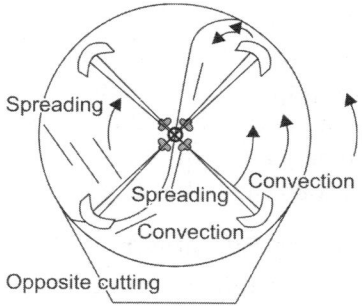

Fig. 9.8: Mechanism of mixing of a double-cone blender

- The mixing barrel can be tilted freely at the angle of 0°~360° for discharging and cleaning purpose.
- The conical shape at both ends enables uniform mixing and easy discharge.
- The cone is statistically balanced to avoid any excessive load on the gear box and motor
- While the powder can be loaded into the cone through a wider opening, it can be discharged through a side valve.
- Depending upon the product, paddle types baffles can be provided on the shaft for better mixing.

6. V-Blenders

It is used for dry mixing. They are totally enclosed to prevent any foreign particles to enter into the chamber. Modifications such as the addition of baffles to increase mixing shear can be done to these type of mixers (Fig. 9.9).

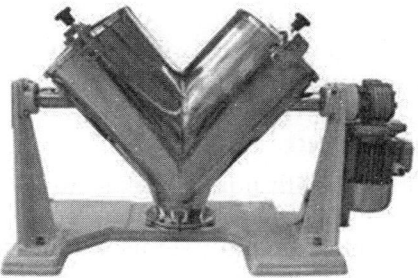

Fig. 9.9: V-Blender

Features

- Minimal attrition when blending fragile granules.
- Large-capacity equipment available.
- It is easier to clean and unload the blender
- Minimal maintenance is required
- Available in various capacities from 25 to 1000 liters.

Tips for Solids Mixing Equipment

1. The proper type of mixer should be chosen to give the desired degree of homogeneity for mixing the materials on hand.
2. Too long a mixing may result in a proper blend. A quantitative relationship between degrees of mixing vs time is worth determining. Except in a few cases, in general, mixing should be over in a few minutes to about 15 minutes if proper equipment is chosen.
3. Care should be taken to prevent or minimize dust formation by using less density but equally effective ingredients or a pellety form of the dusty ingredient, by using dust tight arrangements for loading and unloading the mixer, by addition of liquids like water (where tolerated) along with a trace of surface active agent, etc.
4. Other aspects to be considered are the electrostatic charge, equipment area, contamination of product (from lubricants and repair materials), heating and cooling requirements of the mixer for the problem on hand, flexibility to operate different sized batches (the effect of percent volume occupied by the batch on the adequacy of mixing is to be borne in mind), provision for vacuum or pressure, method of adding liquids, proper ventilation and discharge enclosures, provisions for relief of internal explosion, noise during operation, etc.

SOLID-LIQUID MIXING

The mixing of solid with liquids (i.e. semi-solids) is done for preparing ointments, creams, pill masses and wet mass for making granules, etc. Generally semisolid mixing is carried out in the agitator mixers used for liquids and powders as well as size reduction machines, for example, roller mills, because of the greater consistency, the mixers for semisolids are usually of heavier construction.

Mixers for semi-solids: Mixers for semi-solids are divided into following two:

1. **Agitator mixers**
   a. Sigma mixers, and
   b. Planetary mixers.

2. **Shear mixers**
   a. Colloidal mill, and
   b. Triple roller mill.

Agitator mixers: They are similar in principle to the agitator mixers used for liquids and for powders only the mixers designed specifically for semi-solids are usually of heavier construction to handle materials of greater consistency. The agitator arms are designed to give a pulling and kneading action and the shape and movement is such that material is cleared from all sides and corners of the mixing vessel.

They are of two types, sigma-arm mixer and planetary mixer.

Sigma Mixer

In sigma arm mixer the mixer uses two mixer blades, the shape of which resembles the Greek letter "Sigma". The two blades rotate towards each other and operate in a mixing vessel which has a double trough shape, each blade fitting into a trough. The two blades rotate at different speeds, one usually about twice the speed of the other, resulting in a lateral pulling of the material and division into the two troughs, while the blade shape and difference into the two troughs, while the blade shape and difference in speed causes end-to-end movement. Being of sturdy construction and higher power, this form of mixer can handle even the heaviest plastic materials, and products such as pill masses, tablet granule masses, and ointments are mixed readily. One of the problems encountered in the mixing of semi-solids is the entrainment of air. The mixed product can be easily discharged by tilting the container by hand lever manually either by system of gears manually operated or motorized. The complete mixer is mounted on steel fabricated stand of suitable strength to withstand the vibration and give noise free performance (Fig. 9.10).

The sigma arm mixer can be enclosed and operated under reduced pressure, which is an excellent method for avoiding entrainment of air and may assist in minimizing decomposition of oxidisable materials, but it must be used with caution if the mix contains volatile ingredients.

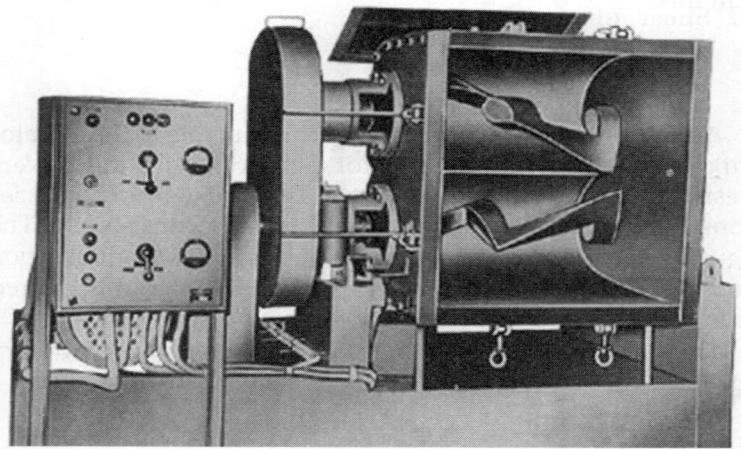

Fig. 9.10: Sigma mixer

The semisolid mixing can be carried out in the agitator mixers meant for mixing liquids and powders. However, the mixers for semisolids are usually of heavier construction. Sigma-arm mixer is the commonly used agitator mixer for the purpose of mixing of semisolids. The mixer has two blades, the shape of which resembles the Greek letter "Sigma" (Fig. 9.11).

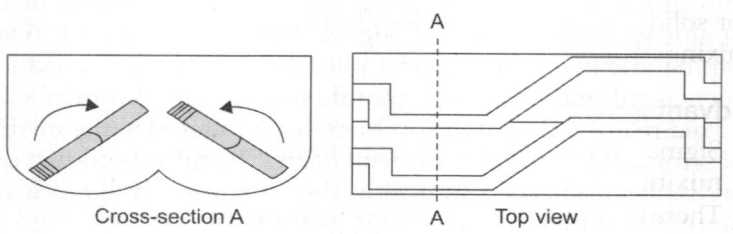

Cross-section A   A   Top view

Fig. 9.11: Agitator (sigma blade) mixer

The two blades move at different speeds and towards each other. The blades operate in a mixing vessel which has a double trough shape, each blade fitted into a trough. The two blades rotate at different speeds, one usually about twice the speed of the other, which causes the lateral pulling of the material and is divided into two troughs. The difference in speed and shape of blades causes end-to-end movement (Fig. 9.12). Air is usually entrapped during the mixing of semisolids. Enclosing the sigma arm mixer and operating it underpressure can avoid this.

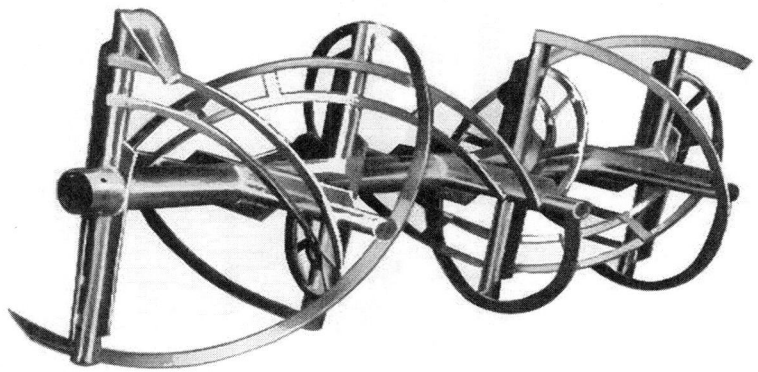

Fig. 9.12: A cross-sectional view of sigma blade

Uses

The sigma-arm mixer is commonly used for mixing of dough ingredient in the baking industry. It is used in wet granulation process in the manufacture of tablets. It is also used for mixing powdered drug with and ointment base. It is primarily used for solid-liquid mixing although it can be used for solid-solid mixing also.

Advantages

• Sigma blade mixer creates a minimum dead space during mixing.
• There is close tolerance between the blades and the sidewalls as well as the bottom of the mixer shell.

Disadvantage

• Sigma mixers work at a fixed speed.

Planetary Mixer

Planetary mixers are used for mixing and beating for viscous and pasty materials, the planetary mixer is still often used for basic operations of mixing and blending in pharmaceutical industry (Fig. 9.13).

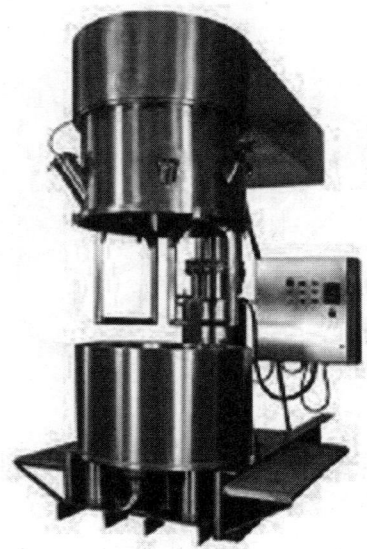

Fig. 9.13: Planetary mixer

Principle: In a planetary mixer, the blade tears the mass apart and shear is applied between a moving blade and a stationary wall. The mixing arm moves around its own axis and also around the central axis in order to reach every spot of the vessel. The plates in the blade are sloped, so that the powder makes an upward movement to produce tumbling motion.

Construction: It consists of a stationary vessel which is made up of stainless steel. The vessel can be removed either by lowering it beneath the blade or raising the blade or raising the blade above the vessel. The mixing blade is mounted from the top of the vessel. The mixing shaft is driven by planetary gear connected to an electric motor. The different types of blades are available for planetary mixer (Fig. 9.14).

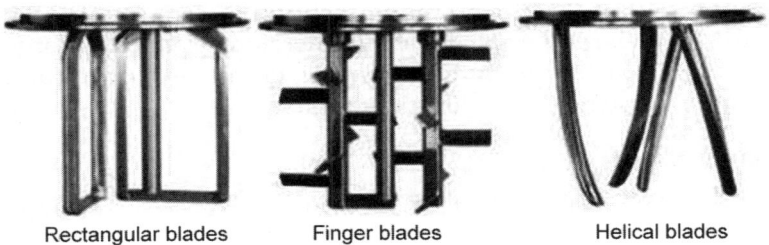

Rectangular blades   Finger blades   Helical blades

Fig. 9.14: Different blade attachment available for planetary mixer

Working: The blade is moved slowly at the initial stage for premixing of the material and finally at increased speed for active missing. In this way high shear can be applied for thorough mixing. The blade and the stationary vessel provide a kneading action and shear. This is due to narrow clearance between the blade and the wall of the vessel.

Uses: The planetary mixer is used for its kneading action required in wet granulation. It is also used for mixing of powdered drug with and ointment base.

Advantage: Planetary mixers work at varying speeds. This is more useful for wet granulation and is advantageous over sigma mixers.

Disadvantages

1. Planetary mixers require high power.
2. Mechanical heat is built up within the powder mix.
3. Use is limited to batch work only

Double Planetary Mixers

The double planetary mixer includes two blades that rotate at their own axis, while they orbit the mix vessel on a common axis. The blades continuously advance along the periphery of the vessel, removing material from the vessel wall and transporting it to the interior. After one revolution the blades have passed through the entire vessel.

Contrary to conventional planetary mixers, the two blade configurations sweep the wall of the vessel clockwise and rotate in opposite directions at about three times the speed of travel. The shear blades displace the material from the walls of the vessel and by their overlapping action the center carry the particles towards the agitator shafts, therefore producing a large field of shear forces. By this means even highly viscous and cohesive material can be efficiently mixed.

Shear Mixer

Machines designed for size reduction can be used for mixing, e.g. roller mills but although the shear forces are good, the general mixing efficiency is poor. Rotary forms may be used and the colloid mill has a stator and a rotor with conical working surfaces. The rotor works at a speed of the order of 3000 to 15000 rpm and the clearance can be adjusted between 50 and 500 micrometers. A roughly mixed suspension or dispersion is introduced through a funnel and is thrown out between the working surfaces by centrifugal force. It is of two types:

1. Colloidal mill (mixer)
2. Triple roller mill (mixer)

1. Colloidal Mill

The colloid mill is useful for milling, dispersing, homogenizing and breaking down of agglomerates in the manufacture of food pastes, emulsions, coatings, ointments, creams, pulps, grease, etc. The main function of the colloid mill is to ensure a breakdown of agglomerates or in the case of emulsions to produce droplets of fine size around 1 micron. The material to be processed is fed by gravity to the hopper or pumped so as to pass between the rotor and stator elements where it is subjected to high shearing and hydraulic forces. Material is discharged through a hopper whereby it can be recirculated for a second pass. For materials having higher solid and fiber contents conical grooved discs are preferred. Sometimes cooling and heating arrangements are also provided in theses mills depending on the type of material being processed. Rotational speed of the rotor varies from 3,000 to 20,000 rpm with the spacing between the rotor and stator capable of very fine adjustment varying from 0.001 to 0.005 inch depending on the size of the equipment. Colloid mills require a flooded feed, the liquid being forced through the narrow clearance by centrifugal action and taking a spiral path. In these mills almost all the energy supplied is converted to heat and the shear forces can unduly increase the temperature of the product. Hence, most colloid mills are fitted with water jackets and it is also necessary to cool the material before and after passing through the mill.

In the premier colloid mill (Fig. 9.15), intense shearing action is produced between the rotor running at several thousand rpm with its working surface in close proximity to the stator. A 5-inch diameter rotor runs at 9000 rpm and has an output of 40–60 gallons depending on the viscosity of the liquid. The gap between the two surfaces is adjustable from 0.3 to 0.002 inch. Crude mix is fed via the hopper to the center of the rotor. The material is flung outward and after homogenization across the shearing surfaces, it is discharged. If the feed is very slow, many hundreds of revolutions will take place while the contents of the gap traverse the working faces and consequently the globules will be subjected to a greater shearing action than effected at the maximum rate of feed (Fig. 9.16). The materials must be supplied at such a rate that the space between the rotor

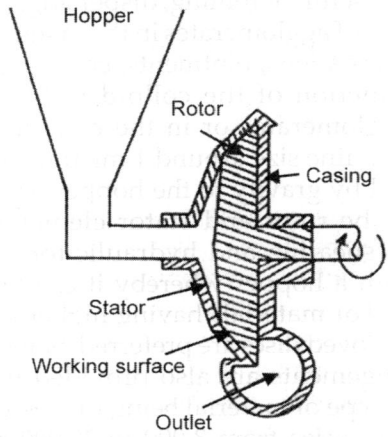

Fig. 9.15: Premier colloid mill (conical grinding surface)

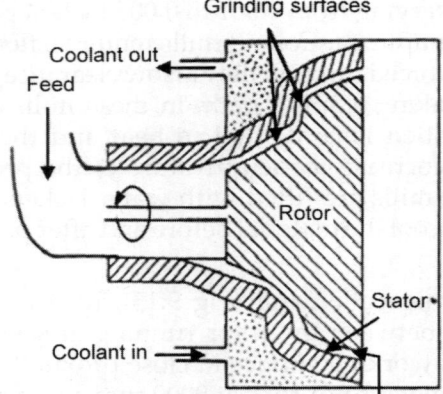

Fig. 9.16: Colloid mill (stepped grinding surface)

and stator is kept entirely filled with liquid. Colloid mills are used in the production of ointment, cream, gels and high viscous fluids for grinding, dispersing and homogenizing in one operation.

Advantages

- Extremely fine particle distribution through optimal shear force.
- High capacity with minimal space requirements.
- Rapid handling and easy cleaning.
- Virtually unlimited application due to highly flexible homogenization system.

2. Triple Roller Mill

Various types of roller mills consisting of one or more rollers are commonly used but triple roller mill is preferred. It is fitted with three rollers which are composed of a hard abrasion-resistant material. They are fitted in such a way that they come in close contact with each other and rotate at different speeds. The material which comes in-between the rollers is crushed and reduced in particle size. The reduction in particle size depends on the gap between the rollers and difference in their speeds.

Construction: The mill consists of three rollers which are made of a hard abrasion-resistant material. These rollers are arranges in such a way that they come very close to each other. These rollers are rotated at different rates of speed. The material coming between the rollers is crushed depending on the gap between them and the difference in rates of movement of the two surfaces (Fig. 9.17).

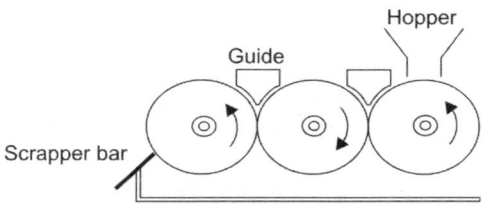

Fig. 9.17: Triple roller mill

Working: As shown the material after passing through hopper, comes between roller 2 and 3 and is reduced in size in the process. The gap between roller 2 and 3 is usually less than that between 1 and 2, further crushed and smoothes the mixture which adheres to roller 2. A scraper is arranged in such a way, that it can remove the mixed material from the roller no. 3 and does not allow the material which has not passed between both sets of the rollers to reach the scraper.

Advantage: The triple roller mill produces very uniform dispersion and is suitable for continuous processes.

Uses: The triple roller mill is very useful for the purpose of mixing of solid powder in ointment base. On large scale, mechanical ointment roller mills are used to obtain an ointment of smooth and uniform texture. The performed coarse ointments are forced to pass through moving stainless steel rollers where it is reduced in particle size and a smooth product which is uniform in composition and texture is obtained. For small-scale work, small ointment mills are available

Material of Construction of Mixers

Materials having sufficient strength and corrosion resistance may be used for the construction of mixers, but stainless steel is favored more for most pharmaceutical applications. Monel metal can be used as an alternative if ferrous metals are to be avoided.

Thus, one can conclude that the process of mixing is one of the most commonly used operations in daily life. A wide variety of materials like liquids, semi-solids and solids require mixing during their formulation into a dosage form, therefore, a proper selection of the mixing equipment is required keeping in mind the physical properties of the materials like density, viscosity, economic considerations regarding processing, i.e. time required for mixing and power requirement and also the cost of the equipment and its maintenance.

PRACTICE QUESTIONS
Very Short Answer Type Questions

1. Discuss in brief the term "mixing".
2. What does the term "perfect mixing" mean?
3. What are the different equipment used for solid-solid mixing?
4. What are the different equipment for mixing of liquid-liquid?
5. What are the different equipment used for mixing of semi-solids?

Short Answer Type Questions

6. What are the various objectives of mixing?
7. Describe briefly different types of mixtures.

Long Answer Type Questions

8. Define the term mixing. Explain the various mechanisms for mixing powders.
9. Enumerate the various physical properties which affect the mixing of powders.
10. Describe the various equipment used for powder mixing.

11. Describe the various equipment used for liquid mixing.

12. Describe the various equipment used for semi-solid mixing?

13. Explain with the help of a neat diagram the construction and working of the following mills:
    a. Triple roller mill
    b. Colloidal mill
    c. Agitated powder mixer
    d. Propeller mixer
    e. Double-cone blender
    f. Planetary mixer

14. Write short notes on:
    a. Colloidal mill
    b. Planetary mixer
    c. Hand mill
    d. Agitator mixer
    e. Double-cone blender

Objective Type Questions

15. Mixing of powders is necessary for preparation of .... , ... and ....

16. Mixing of liquids is done for preparation of .... and ....

17. Mixing of semi-solids is required for preparing ...., ... and ....

18. In agitated powder mixer, mixing of powder takes place, which has .... and ....

19. Match the following:

Column I	Column II
A. The flat blades of paddle mixer rotate at	I. Produces particles in micron size
B. Colloidal mill	II. Rise in temperature
C. Sigma arm mixer	III. 8000 rpm
D. Surface tension decreases with	IV. For mixing of semi-solid
E. The propeller of propeller mixer rotates at	V. 100 rpm

ANSWERS

15. Tablets, capsules and compound powders

16. True solution and emulsions

17. Ointments, creams and pill mass

18. Uniform particle size and density

19. A (V), B (I), C (IV), D (II), E (III)

10

Pharmaceutical Dosage Form

POWDERS

The solid dosage forms are available mostly in unit dosage forms (consisting of doses which are taken by numbers), such as tablets, capsules, pills, cachets or powders. When drugs are to be administered orally in dry state, tablets and capsules are the most convenient dosage form. They are effective and patients have no problem in their handling and administration. Some solids are packed and supplied in bulk powder. The bulk powders meant for external use are dusting powders, insufflations, snuffs and tooth powders. The bulk powders meant for internal use are supplied either as granules or fine powder (Flow chart 10.1).

A pharmaceutical powder is a mixture of finely divided drug and/or chemicals in dry form. These are solid dosage form of medicament which are meant for internal and external use. They are available in crystalline or amorphous form. The particle size of powder plays an important role in physical, chemical and biological properties of the dosage forms. There is a relationship between particle size of powder and dissolution, absorption and therapeutic efficacy of drugs.

Advantages of Powders

1. Powders are one of the oldest dosage form and are used both internally and externally.
2. Powders are more stable than liquid dosage form.
3. It is convenient for the physician to prescribe a specific amount of powdered medicament depending upon the need of the patient.

Flow chart 10.1: Showing various solid dosage form

- Solid dosage forms
  - Unit dosage forms
    - Tablets
      - Oral
      - Lozenge
      - Buccal
      - Sublingual
      - Chewable
      - Soluble
      - Hypodermic
    - Capsules
      - Soft
        - Oral
        - Ointments
      - Hard
    - Suppositories
    - Powders (wrapped)
    - Cachets
      - Dry seal
      - Wet seal
  - Bulk dosage forms
    - For internal use
      - Pills
      - Fine powder
      - Granules
        - Effervescent
        - Non-effervescent
    - For external use
      - Ear powders
      - Ophthalmic powders
      - Tooth powders
      - Snuffs powders
      - Dusting powders

4. The chances of incompatibility are less as compared to liquid dosage form.
5. The onset of action of powdered drug is rapid as compared to other solid dosage form, e.g. tablets, capsules or pills. Due to smaller particle size of powder, it get dissolved easily in body fluids. This rapid dissolution increases the blood concentration in the shorter time and hence the drug action is produces in a shortest period.

Disadvantages of Powders

1. Drugs having bitter, nauseous and unpleasant taste cannot be dispensed in powdered form.
2. Deliquescent and hygroscopic drugs cannot be dispensed in powder form.
3. Drugs which get affected by atmospheric conditions are not suitable for dispensing in powder forms.
4. The dispensing of powder is a time consuming.
5. Quantity less than 100 mg or so, cannot be weighed conveniently on dispensing balance.

Powders solid preparations meant for internal or external use containing one or more drugs mixed with each other in a fine state of subdivision. These are used externally for local application not intended for systemic action. The desired characteristics of powders include (Table 10.1):

1. Homogeneity
2. Non-irritability
3. Free flow
4. Good spreadability and covering capability
5. Adsorption and absorption capacity
6. Very fine state of subdivision
7. Capacity to protect the skin against irritation caused by friction, moisture or chemical irritants.
8. Flow properties of powders
9. Angle of repose
10. Bulk density
11. Carr's index.

$$\text{Carrs index} = \frac{\text{Tapped density} - \text{Poured density}}{\text{Tapped density}}$$

12. Hausner ratio

$$\text{Hausner ratio} = \frac{\text{Tapped density}}{\text{Poured density}}$$

Table 10.1: Characteristics of powder

Flow characteristics	Angle of repose	Carr's index
Very good	<20	5–15
Good	20–30	12–16
OK	25–30	18–21
Poor	30–34	25–35
Very poor		33–38
Extremely poor	>40	>40

CLASSIFICATION OF POWDERS

Powders are classified as
1. Bulk powder for external use
2. Bulk powders for internal use
3. Simple and compound powders
4. Effervescent granules
5. Cachets

1. Bulk Powder for External Use

External bulk powders contain non-potent substances for external applications. These powders are dispensed in glass, plastic wide mouth bottles and also in cardboard with specific method of application. Bulk powders for external used are of following types.
   a. Dusting powders
   b. Snuffs
   c. Douche powders
   d. Dental powders
   e. Insufflation

Dusting Powders

Dusting powders usually contain substances such as zinc oxide, starch and boric acid or natural mineral substances such as kaolin or talc.

Talc may be contaminated with pathogenic microorganisms such as *Clostridium tetani*, etc. and hence it should be sterilized by dry heat. Dusting powders should not be applied to broken skin. If desired, powders should be micronized or passed through a sieve # 80 or 100. Dusting powders should preferably be dispensed in sifter-top containers. Such containers provide the protection from air, moisture and contamination as well as convenience of application. Currently some foot powders and talcum powders have been marketed as pressure aerosols.

Dusting powders are employed chiefly as lubricants, protectives, absorbents, antiseptics, antipruritics, astringents and antiperspirants.

R_x	
Zinc oxide	200 parts
Salicylic acid	20 parts
Starch powder	780 parts (qs)

Snuffs

These are finely divided solid dosage forms of medicaments dispensed in flat metal boxes with hinged lid. These powders are inhaled into nostrils for decongestion, antiseptic, and bronchodilator action.

Douche Powders

These powders are intended to be used as antiseptics or cleansing agents into the body cavity; most commonly for vaginal use although they may be formulated for nasal, otic or ophthalmic use also. As douche powder formation often include aromatic oils, it becomes necessary to pass them through a # 40 or 60 sieve to eliminate agglomeration and to ensure complete mixing. They can be dispended either in wide mouth glass bottles or in powder boxes.

R_x	
Zinc sulphate	2.5 gm
Magnesium sulphate	200 gm
Boric acid	30 gm
Oil of lemon	0.2 gm
Water	1000 ml (qs)

Dental Powders

Dental powders are meant for cleaning the teeth. Dental powders contain detergents, abrasives, antiseptics and coloring and flavoring agents incorporated in a suitable base. Generally the base is calcium carbonate. The detergent is in the form of soap and finely powdered pumice stone provides abrasive action. Essential oils, if present in small quantity, are easily absorbed by calcium carbonate and pumice. This makes the uniform distribution of the oil difficult.

Insufflation

Insufflations are a class of powders meant for application to body cavities, e.g. ear, nose, vagina, etc. The powder has to be extremely fine and must find an entry to the cavity deep enough to bring about its action at the site. It is delivered to the effected part in a stream with the help of the device called an insufflator, which blow the powder to the site. Some of the insufflations contain volatile liquid ingredients which may require uniform distribution in the powder. Active volatile liquid present in small portion should not be removed by evaporation but only incorporated by trituration in the powder. The pharmaceutical industry packages the insufflations in pressurized form, i.e. aerosols. Aerosols contain the medication in a stout container with a suitable valve, the delivery of the powder being accomplished by a liquefied or compressed gas propellant of a very low boiling point. On pressing the actuator of the valve the propellant delivers the medication in a stream.

2. Bulk Powder for Internal Use

Bulk powders contain many doses in a wide-mouth container that is suitable to remove the powder by teaspoon. The non-potent substances are used in bulk powder form such an antacids, laxative, purgative, etc.

R_x	
Rhubarb powder	250 gm
Light magnesium carbonate	325 gm
Heavy magnesium carbonates	325 gm
Ginger powder	100 gm
Make a powder	

3. Simple and Compound Powder for Internal Use

These are unit dose powders normally packed in properly folded papers and dispensed in envelopes, metal foils, small heat-sealed plastic bags or other containers.

Usually for the preparation of simple powders, the ingredients are weighed correctly and blended by geometrical mixing in ascending order of weights. The mixture is then either delivered into blocks of equal size, numbers of blocks representing the number of powder to be dispensed or each dose is weighed separately and placed on a powder paper. The paper is then folded according to the pharmaceutical art and placed in either an envelope or a powder box.

4. Effervescent Granules

This class of preparation can be supplied either by compounding the ingredients as granules or dispensed in the form of salts. The ingredients whether in granular form represent as salts, react in presence of water evolving carbon dioxide gas. For evolution of the gas two constituents are essential, a soluble carbonate such as sodium bicarbonate and an organic acid such as citric or tartaric acid. The preparation can be supplied either as a bulk powder or distributed in individual powders.

There are three alternative methods of dispensing depending upon the nature of prescription.

If the effervescent salts are prescribed to be the dispensed in bulk form, no granulation is necessary. The ingredients are mixed uniformly and directions stated on the label to add the prescribed quantity to water, before use.

1. If the effervescent salt is prescribed in divided doses, the ingredients, which cause effervescence on mixing with water, are enclosed separately in papers of different color and add to the water, before use. Quantities of the sodium bicarbonate and the organic acid, citric or tartaric, are in equimolecular in proportion.

2. In the third case the product contains all the ingredients mixed together in a granular form. Preparation of granular products requires pharmaceutical technique. If sodium bicarbonate and citric acid are taken in equimolecular proportion and mixed to make granules, the quantity of

water of crystallization liberated from the citric acid is large enough to make the mass wet and carbon dioxide may be liberated during the preparation itself. If one tries to substitute citric acid by tartaric acid, which contains no water of crystallization; it may not be possible to form a mass necessary to granulation. Therefore, both citric and tartaric acid are taken in suitable proportion leaving a little acid in surplus than the quantity required to neutralize sodium bicarbonate. This surplus is necessary to give the final preparation an acidic taste that is more palatable. There is a certain loss in weight of such a preparation due to loss of water in drying the granules and partial loss of carbon dioxide due to its release during preparation. Heating is done on a water bath keeping all the ingredients mixed in a porcelain dish. Gentle application of heat liberates the water of crystallization from citric acid and the mass tends to be coherent. The coherent mass is transferred from the porcelain dish and the granules are dried in an oven taking care to regulate the temperature which should be generally kept below 253K. If necessary, the dry granules are passed through a sieve of appropriate size to break larger granules, which result due to sticking of the sieved wet granules.

5. Cachets

Cachet as a unit dosage form was very popular sometime back. Presently cachets are seldom used and have been replaced by capsules. Cachets, like capsules, can be easily filled and sealed at the dispensing counter. This dosage form holds larger quantity of the medication as compared to capsules. Since the cachets are made of flour and water they are easily damaged in handling. Further this dosage form offers a little protection against light and moisture. Due to its size and shape a cachet is difficult to swallow. The process of filling is similar to that of capsules. The drug is placed in one of the two halves of the cachets; the upper half is then placed over it and pressed with the help of a suitable device.

LOZENGES

The word "Lozenge" is derived from French word "Losenge" which means a diamond-shaped geometry having four equal sides. Lozenges are solid preparations that are intended to dissolve in mouth or pharynx. They may contain one or more medicaments in a flavored and sweetened base and are intended to treat local irritation or infection of mouth or pharynx and may also be used for systemic drug absorption. Lozenges are employed for the treatment of local as well systemic disorders. A variety of drug candidates can be incorporated in them for the treatment of and relief from conditions of oral as well as throat infections such as oral thrush, sore throat, cough, gingivitis, pharyngitis, decongestant, etc. Moreover, these also have been used to deliver the drug systemically for smoking cessation and pain relief. Though the lozenge dissolution time is about 30 minutes, it also depends on the patient, as patient controls the rate of dissolution and absorption by sucking on lozenge until it dissolves. The consequence of this can be high variabilities in amounts of drug delivered each time the lozenge is administered. Depending on the type of lozenge, they may be prepared by molding or by compression. Molded lozenges are called pastilles while compressed lozenges are called troches.

Lozenges should dissolve slowly in mouth and possess some degree of smoothness, with their shape being without corners. Lozenges may be formulated with various shapes, like flat, circular, octagonal, biconvex or bacilli, meaning short rods or cylinders. Most of the lozenge formulations are available as over-the-counter (OTC) products where there is no need of prescription from a medical practitioner while some are prescribed by the medical practitioners.

Advantages

a. Can be given to those patients who have difficulty in swallowing.

b. Easy to administer to geriatric and pediatric population.

c. Has a pleasant taste.

d. It extends the time of drug in the oral cavity to elicit a specific effect.

e. Easy to prepare, with minimum amount of equipment and time.

f. Do not require water intake for administration.

g. Technique is non invasive, as is the case with parenterals.

Disadvantages

a. It could be mistakenly taken as candy by children, hence should be kept out of the reach of children.
b. Possible draining of drug from oral cavity to stomach along with saliva.

Lozenges currently available in market are of four types

1. Caramel based medicated lozenges
2. Compressed tablet lozenges
3. Soft lozenges, and
4. Hard candy lozenges

Caramel Based or Chewy Medicated Lozenges

These are the dosage form in which medicament is incorporated into a caramel base which is chewed instead of being dissolved in mouth. It consist of a mixture of sugar and corn syrup in a ratio of 50 : 50 to 75 : 25 sugar to corn syrup. Whipping agent like milk protein, egg albumin, gelatin are used to incorporate air in toffee-based confections to obtain the desired degree of soft chew. Humectants like glycerin, propylene glycol and sorbitol are added to improve chew and mouthfeel properties. The medicaments up to 35–40% can be incorporated.

Manufacturing

The candy base is cooked at 95–125°C and transferred to planetary or sigma blade mixer. Mass is allowed to cool to 120°C. This is followed by the addition of whipping agent below 105°C. The medicaments are then added between 95 and 105°C. Color is dispersed in humectant and added to the above mass at a temperature above 90°C. Seeding crystals and flavor are then added below 85°C followed by lubricant addition above 80°C.

Compressed Tablet Lozenges

If the active ingredient is heat labile, it may be made into lozenge preparation by compression. The granulation is prepared in a manner similar to that used for any compressed tablet. The lozenge tablets differ from conventional tablets in terms of organolepticity, non-disintegrating characteristics and slower dissolution profiles. The lozenge is made using heavy compression equipment to give a tablet that is harder than usual, as it is desirable for the troche to dissolve slowly in mouth. They are usually flat faced with Sizes,weight , hardness and erosion time ranging between 3/4 inch, 1.5–4 gm, 30–50 kg/m and 5–10 minutes respectively.

Manufacturing

Direct compression—ingredients can be thoroughly mixed and directly compressed.

Wet granulation—in this sugar is pulverized by mechanical comminution to a fine powder (40–80 mesh).

Medicament is added and the mass is blended mass. The blended is subjected to granulation with sugar or corn syrup and screened through 2–8 mesh screen. This is followed by drying and milling to 10–30 mesh size. Flavor and lubricant are then added prior to the compression.

Soft Lozenges

Soft lozenges are either meant for chewing or for slow dissolution in mouth.

They can be made from PEG 1000 or 1450, chocolate or sugar-acacia base while some soft lozenge formulations can also contain acacia and silica gel. Acacia is used to provide texture and smoothness to the lozenge and silica gel is used as a suspending agent to avoid settling of materials to the bottom of the mold cavity during the cooling. The formulation requires heating process at about 50°C hence is only suitable to heat-resistant ingredients.

Manufacturing

On the account of the soft texture of these lozenges, they can be hand rolled and then cut into pieces or the warm mass can be poured into a plastic mold. Mold cavity should be overfilled if PEG is used, as PEG's contract as they cool. This is not required in case of chocolate as it does not shrink.

Hard Candy Lozenges

Hard candy lozenges are mixtures of sugar and other carbohydrates in an amorphous (noncrystalline) or glassy state.

They can also be regarded as solid syrups of sugars. The moisture content and weight of hard candy lozenge should be between, 0.5 to 1.5% and 1.5–4.5 gm respectively. These should undergo a slow and uniform dissolution or erosion over 5–10 min, and should not disintegrate. The temperature requirements for their preparation is usually high hence heat labile materials cannot be incorporated in them.

Packaging

Since the lozenges are hygroscopic in nature a complex and multiple packaging is adopted. The individual unit is wrapped in polymeric moisture barrier material which are then placed in tight or moisture resistant glass, polyvinyl chloride or metal container that is over wrapped by aluminum foil or cellophane membrane.

Storage

Lozenges should be stored away from heat and out of reach of children. They should be protected from extremes of humidity. Depending upon the storage requirements of both, the drug and the base, either room temperature or refrigerator temperature is usually indicated.

LIQUID DOSAGE FORM

Liquid dosage forms commonly used in pharmaceutical practice are either monophasic or biphasic. Monophasic systems are characterized by the presence of a single homogeneous phase, e.g. solution, mixtures, elixirs, tinctures, syrups, ear drop, nasal drops, etc. whereas biphasic liquid dosage forms consist of two distinct phases, e.g. emulsions and suspensions. Liquid preparations may be broadly classified under two categories (Flow chart 10.2).

1. Internal Liquid Preparation

A. Monophasic liquid preparations
  a. Syrups
  b. Elixirs
  c. Solutions
  d. Linctuses

Flow chart 10.2: Various liquid dosage form

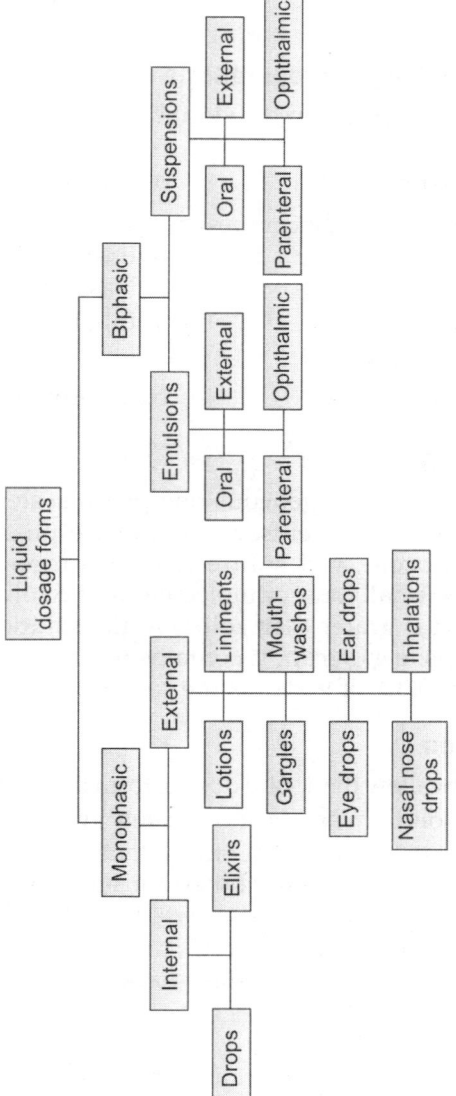

B. Biphasic liquid preparations
   a. Suspension (mixture)
   b. Emulsion

2. External Liquid Preparations

A. Topical (applied on the skin)
   a. Lotions   b. Liniments
   c. Throat paints   d. Collodions

B. Instilled into body cavities
   a. Douches   b. Enemas
   c. Ear drops   d. Nasal drops
   e. Nasal sprays   f. Inhalations

C. Used in mouth
   a. Gargles   b. Mouthwashes

SOLUTIONS

A solution is a homogeneous one-phase system consisting of two or more components. Solvent is the phase in which the dispersion occur and solute is that components which is dispersed is small ions or molecules in the solvent. In general, solvent part is grater than solute in the solution except a few preparations, e.g. syrup, it contains 66.7% w/w of sucrose as solute and 33.3% of water as the solvent.

Advantages

- Easy to swallow than solid dosage form like tablet and capsules.
- Drug in solution form is immediately available for absorption.
- A solution is a homogeneous system and therefore the drug remains uniformly distributed throughout the preparation.
- Suitable for drugs that can irritate and damage the gastric mucosa, if localized in a specific area. The irritation is reduced by administration in solution form.

Disadvantages

- Inconvenient to transport and store because they are bulky.
- Whole product is lost immediately if any breakage in the container.
- The stability of most of substances in aqueous solution is less than solid dosage form.

- Self life of solution is shorter than solid preparation
- Suitable media for the microbial contamination and may therefore require suitable preservatives.
- Dose inaccuracy compared to solid dosage form.
- Bitter unpleasant substance are not suitable for solutions and need sweetening and flavoring agent to make them more palatable.

Method of Preparation

Following additives are generally required for preparation of solution

- **Solvents**
  - a. Aqueous
  - b. Non-aqueous (fixed oil, alcohol, polyhydric alcohol, dimethyl-sulphoxide, ethyl ether, liquid paraffin, etc.
- **Buffers:** Carbonates, citrates, gluconates, lactates, phosphate, tartrate, borates, etc.
- **Colors:** Water soluble dye amaranth.
- Density modifiers.
- Flavors and perfumes.
- Taste enhancer.
  - *a. Salty:* Apricot, butterscotch, liquorice, peach, vanilla.
  - *b. Bitter:* Anise, chocolate, mint, wild cherry.
  - *c. Sweet:* Vanilla fruits.
  - *d. Sour:* Citrus fruits, raspberry.
- Preservatives.
- Antioxidants and reducing agents.

Container

Narrow mouth, screw capped, colorless plain bottle and amber colored bottle for heat sensitive drugs.

Example: Prepare and dispense cresol with soap solution

R_x	
Cresol	500 ml
Vegetable oil	180 gm
Potassium hydroxide	42 gm
Purified water, sufficient to produce	1000 ml

Method of dispensing: Dissolve potassium hydroxide in purified water (50%), add vegetable oil and heat on a water-bath and mix thoroughly. Continue heating until a small portion dissolved in water without separation of oily drops. Add cresol and mix thoroughly with sufficient purified water.

Example: Prepare and dispense aqueous iodine solution (Lugol's solution)

R_x	
Iodine	50 gm
Potassium iodide	100 gm
Purified water	1000 ml

Method of dispensing: Dissolve potassium iodide and iodine in purified water and mix thoroughly. Finally make up the volume with the help of purified water.

Example: Prepare and dispense strong iodine solution

R_x	
Iodine	100 gm
Potassium iodide	60 gm
Purified water	100 ml
Ethanol, sufficient to produce	1000 ml

Method of dispensing: Dissolve potassium iodide and iodine in purified water and add sufficient ethanol to make up the volume.

Example: Prepare and dispense weak iodine solution

R_x	
Iodine	20 gm
Potassium iodide	25 gm
Purified water	100 ml
Ethanol, sufficient to produce	1000 ml

Method of dispensing: Dissolve potassium iodide and iodine in purified water. Add sufficient ethanol to produce 1000 ml.

MIXTURES

A mixture is a liquid preparation meant for oral administration in which medicament or medicaments are dissolved or suspended in a suitable vehicle. Generally, several doses are dispensed in a bottle. In case, a bottle contains one dose, it is called draught. Mixtures differs from solution that the mixture may be homogeneous or heterogeneous are for oral administration whereas solution are homogeneous and are for external or internal use. Mixtures are not prepared to keep them for a long period because they are mainly prescribed for acute conditions such as cough, indigestion, diarrhea, constipation, etc. So the mixtures should be extemporaneously prepared and supplied only for small number of doses which can be used up within a short period. In case further need arises, then a fresh mixture is prepared for the patient.

Advantages

1. They are more effective than solid dosage forms.
2. Certain substances can be only given in liquid because they are inconvenient to administer in any other form, e.g. castor oil, liquid paraffin.
3. Mixtures are easy to administer and economical compare to other dosage form.

Disadvantages

1. They are comparatively less stable than solid dosage forms.
2. They are more bulky and difficult to carry.

Classification of mixtures: Mixtures are classified into:

1. Simple mixture containing soluble substances
2. Mixtures containing diffusible solids
3. Mixtures containing indiffusible solids
4. Mixtures containing precipitates forming liquids
5. Mixtures containing slightly soluble liquids

1. Simple mixtures containing soluble substances: Simple mixtures contains only soluble ingredients, e.g. carminative mixture, diarrhea mixture and expectorant mixture.

Example: *Dispense 900 ml of the mixture.*

R_x	
Potassium bromide	40 gm
Tincture nux vomica	40 ml
Chloroform water	900 ml (qs)

1. Mixtures containing diffusible solids: Diffusible solids are those which do not dissolve in water, but may be mixed there with so that, upon shaking, the powder drug is evenly diffused throughout the liquid for sufficient time to ensure uniform distribution in each dose. The commonly used diffusible drugs are bismuth carbonate, bismuth subnitrate, magnesium carbonate (heavy or light), magnesium oxide (heavy or light), quinine sulphate, light kaolin, etc.

Example: *Dispense the following mixture.*

R_x	
Magnesium sulphate	150 gm
Magnesium carbonate	20 gm
Peppermint water	900 ml (qs)
Prepare a mixture	

1. Mixtures containing indiffusible solids: Indiffusible solids are those solids which are not soluble in water and do not soluble in water and do not remain uniformly distributed in the vehicle for sufficiently long time. Therefore, to suspend the drug, suspending agents are added. The commonly used indiffusible drugs in mixtures form are acetyl salicylic acid, quinine salicylate, calomel, phenacetin, benzoic acid, phenobarbitone prepared chalk, etc.

The suspending agents which are commonly used in mixtures containing indiffusible solids are:

    a. Compound tragacanth powder: In the proportion of 2 gm/100 ml (10 grains-ounce) of the mixture.

    b. Tragacanth mucilage: In the proportion of 1/4th or the volume of the mixture.

Mixture containing precipitate forming liquids: Certain liquid preparation contain resinous matter, when mixed with water, the resin is precipitated which may adhere to the sides of the bottle or form a clotted precipitate which will not re-diffuse upon shaking. To prevent this compound tragacanth powder or tragacanth mucilage are used (Tables 10.2 and 10.3).

Table 10.2: Comparison between mixture and pure compound

Mixtures	Pure compounds
A mixture can be physically separated into pure compounds or elements.	A pure compound has a constant composition with fixed ratios of elements
Mixtures exhibit physical properties which are not fixed. For example, mixture of alcohol and water boils over a range of temperatures	Physical properties such as boiling point or melting point of pure substances are fixed. For example, pure water boils at 100°C

Table 10.3: Comparison between homogeneous mixture and hetero-geneous mixture

Homogeneous mixtures	Heterogeneous mixtures
The prefixes "homo"—indicate sameness	The prefixes: "hetero"—indicate difference
A homogeneous mixture has the same uniform appearance and composition throughout. Many homogeneous mixtures are commonly referred to as solutions	A heterogeneous mixture consists of visibly different substances or phases. The three phases or states of matter are gas, liquid, and solid.
Particle size distinguishes homogeneous solutions from other heterogeneous mixtures. Solutions have particles which are the size of atoms or molecules—too small to be seen, e.g. a **colloid** is a homogeneous solution	In contrast a **suspension** is a heterogeneous mixture of larger particles. These particles are visible and will settle out on standing. Examples of suspensions are: Fine sand or silt in water or tomato juice
Corn oil is homogeneous, white vinegar is homogeneous. A sugar solution is homogeneous since only a colorless liquid is observed. Air with no clouds is homo-geneous	For example, beach sand is heterogeneous. Vinegar and oil salad dressing is heterogeneous since two liquid layers are present, as well as solids. Air with clouds is heterogeneous, as the clouds contain tiny droplets of liquid water

SPIRITS

Spirits are alcoholic or hydroalcoholic preparations containing volatile substances. The volatile ingredient may be in the form of solid, liquid or gas. They are generally used for internally as well as externally as inhalations for their medicinal value while there major use is as flavoring agent. They may be used in the formulation of aromatic waters or as pharmaceutical aids. Brandy (spirits invites) and whisky (spiritus frumenti) and ends with a wide variety of products that comply with the definition given above. Physicians have debated the therapeutic value of the formed products and these are no longer official in the compendia. The BP, definition of spirits is very broad. Some examples are aromatic ammonia spirits BP, which has different formula from the USP XXI, is used as a flavoring agent. Soap spirits BP is used instead of a shampoo for scalp disorders and surgical spirits BP is used for the astringent action on unbroken skin.

Methylated spirits ("metho") is a mixture of ethyl alcohol (95%) and methyl alcohol (5%). The methyl alcohol is poisonous and is added to prevent the methylated spirits being used as cheap drinking alcohol. Methyl alcohol, or methanol, is also sometimes called wood spirit. It is produced by the destructive distillation of wood, or by a synthetic process which involves reacting carbon monoxide with hydrogen gas. It is poisonous and, if consumed, causes blindness, insanity, and eventual death. It is commonly used as a denaturant for ethyl alcohol, and is miscible with water.

Storage: Spirits should be stored in tight, light-resistant containers and in a cool place. This tends to prevent evaporation and volatilization of either the alcohol or the active principal and to limit oxidative changes, spirits usually contain a high alcohol content and consequently should be kept away from an open flame.

Method of Preparation of Spirits

It is prepared by following methods
1. Simple solution
2. Solution with maceration
3. Chemical reaction
4. Distillation

1. **Simple solution:** It is the simplest procedure in which the volatile substance is dissolved in alcohol. Sometimes filtered to obtain a clear solution. Examples are ether spirit, chloroform spirit, peppermint spirit.

2. **Solution with maceration:** In this method leaves of drugs are macerated in purified water to extract water soluble constituents. The marc is pressed and expressed liquid is mixed with the extract. Then sufficient quantity of alcohol is added and the liquid is filtered. Official peppermint is prepared while peppermint spirit BPC is prepared by dissolving peppermint in alcohol only.

3. **Chemical reaction:** None of the official spirits are prepared by this method.

4. **Distillation:** Aromatic spirit of ammonia IP is prepared by this method, in this method distillation unit is used for the preparation of spirit. The methods involve distillation of leaves of drugs soaked in purified water in the round bottom flask which is subjected to distillation. Finally after passing through the condenser the distillate is obtained in another flask.

Example: Prepare and dispense chloroform spirit IP.

R_x	
Chloroform	50 ml
Alcohol (90%)	1000 ml (qs)

Method of dispensing: Mix chloroform with small quantity of alcohol, shake it for some time and finally add more alcohol to make up the volume.

Storage: Stored in a well-closed container in a cool and dark place. Since chloroform converts to phosgene in presence of air and sunlight hence it is to be stored in amber color bottle and the solution is filled up to the brim.

Example: Prepare and dispense peppermint spirit IP.

R_x	
Peppermint oil	100 ml
Alcohol (90%)	1000 ml (qs)

Method of dispensing: Dissolve peppermint oil in small quantity of alcohol, shake it for some time and finally add more alcohol to make up the volume. If the solution is not clear to this add 50 gm of purified talc and shake, set aside for some time and then filter to get the clear solution.

Storage: Stored in a well-closed container in a cool and dark place.

AROMATIC WATERS

Aromatic waters are saturated solutions unless otherwise specified of volatile oils or other aromatic or volatile substances in distilled water. They are clear and free from solid impurities. They possess an odor similar to the plant or volatile substance from which they are made, and are free from impurities or foreign odors. Aromatic waters should be protected from strong light and preferably stored in containers which are stoppered with purified cotton to allow access of some air but to exclude dust.

Aromatic waters are prepared by one of the following processes.

1. **Distillation:** Place the odoriferous portion of the plant or drug from which the aromatic water is to be prepared in a suitable still with sufficient water, and distil most of the water, carefully avoiding the development of odors through the burning of the substances. Separate any excess of oil, and preserve or use the clear aqueous portion, which should be saturated with the flavoring or aromatic principles of the plant. Examples are chloroform water, camphor water, cinnamon water, etc.

2. **Solution:** The volatile oil, or other specified volatile substance, 2 cc or 2 gm; distilled water, a sufficient quantity, to make 1000 cc. Shake the volatile substance with 1000 cc of distilled water in a capacity bottle, and repeat the shaking several times during a period of about fifteen minutes. Set the mixture aside for twelve hours for overnight, filter through paper, and pass enough distilled water through the filter to obtain 1000 cc.

   If preferred, the aromatic water may be prepared by the above formula but with the addition of about 15 gm of purified talc, or a sufficient quantity of purified siliceous earth, or pulped filter paper, with which the volatile substance is thoroughly incorporated. Agitate the mixture well, and filter, until a clear solution is obtained after filtration.

3. **Dilution method:** In this method aromatic water I prepared by diluting the concentrated water with 39 times its volume of purified water. Aromatic water prepared by this method usually contains 1.5% of (90%) alcohol.

Example: Prepare and dispense chloroform water IP.

R_x	
Chloroform	2.5 ml
Purified water	1000 ml (qs)

Method of dispensing: Chloroform is added to purified water, the resulting solution is shaken vigorously for 30 minutes. The shaking is done in a closed vessel because chloroform is volatile.

Storage: Stored in a well-closed container in a cool and dark place.

Example: Prepare and dispense camphor water IP

R_x	
Camphor	1 gm
Alcohol (90%)	2 ml
Purified water	1000 ml (qs)

Method of dispensing: Dissolve the camphor in alcohol, add the solution in successive portions to the purified water. Shake well for 30 minutes.

Storage: Stored in a well-closed container in a cool and dark place.

GLYCERIN

Glycerin is a chemical compound also commonly called glycerol or glycerin. It is a colorless, odorless, viscous liquid that is widely used in pharmaceutical formulations. For human consumption, glycerol is classified by the FDA among the sugar alcohols as a caloric macronutrient.

In foods and beverages, glycerin serves as a humectant, solvent and sweetener, and may help preserve foods. It is also used as filler in commercially prepared low-fat foods (e.g. cookies), and as a thickening agent in liquors. Glycerol also serves as a way, along with water, to preserve certain types of leaves. Glycerol is also used as a sugar substitute. In this regard, it has approximately 27 calories per teaspoon and is 60% as sweet as sucrose. Although it has about the same food energy as table sugar, it does not raise blood sugar levels, nor does it feed the bacteria that form plaques and cause dental cavities.

Glycerin is also used to manufacture mono- and di-glycerides for use as emulsifiers, as well as polyglycerol esters going into shortenings and margarines.

Pharmaceutical and Personal Care Applications

Glycerol is used in medical and pharmaceutical and personal care preparations, mainly as a means of improving smoothness, providing lubrication and as a humectant. It is found in cough syrups, elixirs and expectorants, toothpaste, mouthwashes, skin care products, shaving cream, hair care products, soaps and water based personal lubricants.

As a 10% solution, glycerol prevents tannins from precipitating in ethanol extracts of plants (tinctures). It is also used as a substitute for ethanol as a solvent in preparing herbal extractions. It is less extractive and is approximately 30% less able to be absorbed by the body. Fluid extract manufacturers often extract herbs in hot water before adding glycerin to make glycerites.

Used as a laxative when introduced into the rectum in suppository or liquid (enema) form; irritates the bowel and induces a hyperosmotic effect.

Glycerol is a component of glycerol soap, which is made from denatured alcohol, glycerol, sodium castorate (from castor), sodium cocoate, sodium tallowate, sucrose, water, and fragrance. Sometimes one adds sodium laureth sulfate. This kind of soap is used by people with sensitive, easily-irritated skin because it prevents skin dryness with its moisturizing properties. It is possible to make glycerol soap at home.

It is also used in de-/anti-icing fluids, as in vitrification of blood cells for storage in liquid nitrogen.

In motion-picture production, glycerol is used as a non-evaporating substitute for perspiration on actors. It is also used in the formulation of some types of stage blood.

PAINTS

Throat paints are viscous liquid preparations used for mouth and throat infections. Glycerin is commonly used as a base because being viscous, it adheres to mucous membrane for a long period. It also provides a sweet taste to the preparation. The commonly used throat paints are boroglycerin, phenol glycerin, tannic acid glycerin, compound iodine paint (mandl's paint).

Paints are solution or dispersions of one or more medicaments intended for application to the skin or, in some cases to the mucous membrane. They may contain volatile solvent that evaporates quickly to leave a dry or resinous film of medicament. Throat paints are more viscous due to high content of glycerin. Paints are sticky and adhere to the affected site and prolong the action of the medicament. Common example of paste are:

1. Brilliant green and crystal violet paints
2. Crystal violet paints
3. Coal tar paints
4. Mandl's paint
5. Tannic acid glycerin paints.

Storage: Paint should be kept in airtight containers.

Label: It should state "For external use only". Away from sunlight.

Container: "In a wide mouth screw capped bottles".

Example: Prepare and dispense brilliant green and crystal violet paint.

R_x	
Brilliant green	5 gm
Crystal violet	5 gm
Ethanol	500 ml
Purified water	1000 ml (qs)

Method of dispensing: Dissolve the brilliant green and crystal violet in ethanol (90%) add sufficient water to produce 1000 ml.

Example: Prepare and dispense crystal violet paints.

R_x	
Crystal violet	1 gm
Purified water	1000 ml (qs)

Method of dispensing: Disperse the crystal violet in 700 ml of water and allow it to stand for one hour filter if necessary and make up the volume with water to 1000 ml.

Example: Prepare and dispense iodine paints (Mandl's paint)

In this preparation iodine act as antiseptic and potassium iodide dissolve the iodine, peppermint oil act as flavoring agent and produce cooling effect, alcohol is used as a solubilizing agent for the peppermint oil. This preparation contains iodine, hence should be prepared id glass apparatus. It should not be prepared in mortar and pestle because porcelain contains pores and iodine enters in these pores. It is difficult to wash out the iodine and this entangled iodine can change the color of other preparations.

R_x	
Potassium iodide	25 gm
Iodine	125 gm
Ethanol (90%)	40 ml
Peppermint oil	4 ml
Purified water	25 ml
Glycerin	1000 ml (qs)

Method of dispensing: Dissolve potassium iodide and iodine in purified water in glass mortar and pestle with small portion of glycerin, add peppermint oil, dissolve in ethanol and mix. Add sufficient glycerin to produce 1000 ml.

SYRUPS

Syrups are concentrated oral solutions of sugar or nearly saturated solutions of sucrose in water or other aqueous liquids.

Syrups containing 85% w/v or 66.7% w/w sucrose will retard the growth of microorganisms. Dilute solution of sucrose provides an excellent nutritional media for the growth of yeast, moulds and other microorganisms. When heat is employed for the preparation of syrups, a small portion of sucrose changes to dextrose and levulose. This phenomenon is called inversion. Sucrose solution is optically active and rotates polarized light to right while on heating optical activity decreases rotated the light to left due to formation of other compounds (dextrose ad levulose). The rate of inversion is enhanced by the presence of acids and hydrogen ions, which act as catalyst.

Syrups are mainly of three types

1. **Simple syrup:** It contains sucrose in purified water alone or in combination of other polyols such as glycerin or sorbitol. These substances are added in syrups to reduce the crystallization of sucrose or improve the solubility of excipients.

2. **Medicated syrup:** It contains some added medicinal substances in the syrups and used for therapeutic purpose, e.g. ephedrine sulphate syrup.

3. **Flavored syrup:** It contains various aromatic or pleasantly flavored substances but are non-medicated and generally used as vehicle or as a flavoring agent or for preservation.

Methods of Preparation

Preparation of syrup depends on the physical and chemical characteristics of the substance employed for its preparation of syrups.

1. **Agitation without heat:** This method is used for the preparation of syrups containing volatile substances. In this process active medicament is added in solution and mixed in a glass-stopper bottle. For preparing large quantities, glass lined tank with mechanical agitators is employed. This method is used for the preparation of wide variety of syrups. Cough syrups are commonly prepared by this process, e.g. codeine syrup, ephedrine sulfate syrup, etc.

2. **Solution with heat:** This process is generally preferred as it is simple and less time consuming method, particularly if the constituents are not affected by heat and are non-volatile in nature. In this process sucrose is added in the aqueous solution and heated till the sucrose is dissolved completely. Adding remaining amount of distilled water makes up volume of the solution. If the syrups containing any substances which are coagulated, it can be separated subsequently by straining. Excessive heating of syrup is not suitable because more inversion of sucrose occurs with the increase in temperature. Syrups cannot be sterilized in autoclave without caramelization. This solution is converted in yellowish to brown color due to formation of caramel by the effect of heat on sucrose.

3. **Addition of a medicated liquid:** This method is used when other medicated substances in liquid form are added to syrup to medicate it. In this process some time precipitation takes place due to the presence of resinous and oily substances. It is necessary to take care that medicated substance should not get precipitated in this process.

4. **Percolation:** In this process, purified water or an aqueous solution is allowed to pass through a bed of crystalline sucrose. A plug of cotton is put in the neck of the percolator and purified water or aqueous solution is added in the percolator containing sucrose. The flow rate is controlled by the stopcock and maintained such that drops appear in rapid succession. If required, a small portion of liquid is re-passed through the percolator to dissolve the sugar completely in the liquid or aqueous solvent.

Preservatives

Syrup should be kept at low temperature, about 25°C is suitable for preservation. Preservatives are used to prevent bacterial and mould growth, viz. methyl paraben, proply paraben, sodium benzoate, benzoic acid, etc.

Label and Storage

Syrup should be kept in well-closed containers and stored at temperature below 30°C. Bottle should be completely filled, carefully stoppered and stored in a cool and dark place.

Example: Prepare and dispense simple syrup.

R_x	
Sucrose	667 gm
Purified water, sufficient to produce	1000 gm

Or

R_x	
Sucrose	850 gm
Purified water, sufficient to produce	1000 ml

Example: Prepare and dispense invert syrup.

R_x	
Sucrose	66.7 gm
Purified water, sufficient to produce	100.0 gm
Hydrochloric acid	qs
Sodium carbonate as neutralizing agent	

Method of dispensing: Prepare syrup of sucrose 66.6% w/w in purified water and add hydrochloric acid slowly with continuous stirring. Neutralize the solution using sodium carbonate solution

Example: Prepare and dispense tolu syrup (1000 ml).

R_x	
Tolu balsam	12.5 gm
Sucrose	660 gm
Purified water	1000 ml qs

Method of dispensing: Boil 400 ml of purified water in a vessel. Add weighed amount of tolu balsam in boiled water cover the vessel partially and boil the contents for 30 minutes. With frequently stirring add purified water to make contents of the vessel about to 360 gm. Cool it and filter the solution add sucrose in the solution and warm it on a water bath to dissolve sucrose completely. Add sufficient water to make 1000 ml of the solution.

ELIXIRS

Elixirs are clear, flavored hydroalcoholic preparation intended for oral use. They contain one or more medicament, pleasantly flavored usually attractively colored containing high proportion of alcohol or sucrose along with some suitable antimicrobial agent. The alcoholic content in elixir vary from 5–40%. In general they are more stable than mixture as sufficient alcohol is added to maintain the drug in the solution.

Elixirs are of Two Types

1. **Non-medicated elixirs:** They are used purely as diluting agents or solvents for drugs containing approximately 25% alcohol, e.g. simple elixirs is alcoholic elixirs or low alcohol elixirs (containing 7–10% alcohol) and high alcoholic elixirs (containing 60–75% alcohol).

2. **Medicated elixirs:** Elixirs containing therapeutically active compounds are known as medicated elixirs, e.g. phenobarbital elixirs USP, dexamethasone elixirs USP chlorpheniramine maleate elixirs.

The elixirs are generally marketed as ready to use like cough syrups, viz. dextromethorphan hydrobromide, codeine phosphate ammonium chloride some elixirs (phenethicillin and phenoxymethyl penicillin) are available in the market in granule or powder form because active ingredients are unstable in solution and there constituent will get degraded in presence of water. Hence, they are labeled as "Make up the volume up to the mark and shake well before use". The label also contain "store in a cool and dark place" and used the constituents within one week.

Example: Prepare and dispense high alcohol elixir.

R_x	
Compound orange spirit	4 ml
Saccharin	3 ml
Glycerin	200 ml
Alcohol	1000 ml (qs)

Method of dispensing: Dissolve the compound orange spirit and the saccharin in 70.0 ml of alcohol and glycerin. Add sufficient amount of alcohol to produce 100.0 ml and mix properly. Filter the mixture and preserve in suitable container.

Example: Prepare and dispense simple elixir.

R_x	
Orange tincture	75 ml
Syrup	400 ml
Chloroform water	1000 ml (qs)

Method of dispensing: Mix orange tincture with the syrup and add sufficient chloroform water to produce 100.0 ml. Add 5% of purified talc and shake vigorously. Filter the elixir and preserve in a sutaible container.

Example: Prepare and dispense pediatric paracetamol elixir.

R_x	
Paracetamol	24 ml
Ethanol (96%)	100 ml
Propylene glycol	100 ml
Concentrated raspberry juice	25 ml
Chloroform spirit	20 ml
Invert syrup	275 ml
Amaranth solution	2 ml
Glycerin	1000 ml (qs)

Method of dispensing: Mix ethanol (96%), propylene glycol and chloroform spirit and make a mixture. Dissolve paracetamol and shake it, add other additives. Finally sufficient amount of glycerin to produce 1000 ml.

Example: Prepare terpin hydrate elixir.

R_x	
Terpin hydrate	50 gm
Orange oil	0.2 ml
Glycerin	400 ml
Alcohol	425 ml
Syrup	100 ml
Purified water	1000 ml (qs)

Method of dispensing: Dissolve terpin hydrate in alcohol and add other additives. Add sufficient purified water to produce 100 ml and mix if necessary, filter the elixir and preserve in a suitable container.

MOUTHWASHES

A mouthwash is an aqueous solution which is most often used for its deodorant, refreshing or antiseptic effect. It may contain alcohol, glycerin, synthetic sweeteners, surface-active agent, flavoring and coloring agents. Mouthwashes generally contain following substances.

1. **Antibacterial agents:** Alkaline phenol, hydrogen peroxide, buffered sodium perborate, thymol glycerin.
2. **Astringents:** Zinc sulphate, zinc chloride, etc.

Container: Narrow mouthed screw-capped colored fluted bottle.

Label: The label on the container should state—"Not to be swallowed in larges amount" and "Stored in a cool and dark place away from sunlight".

Example: Prepare and dispense compound sodium chloride mouthwash.

R_x	
Sodium bicarbonate	10 gm
Sodium chloride	15 gm
Concentrated peppermint emulsion	25 ml
Double strength chloroform water	500 ml
Purified water qs	1000 ml

Method of dispensing: Dissolve sodium bicarbonate and sodium chloride in purified water, add concentrated peppermint emulsion and mix. Add double strength chloroform water. Finally make up the volume with purified water.

Example: Prepare and dispense mouthwash.

R_x	
Cetylpyridinium chloride	1 gm
Citric acid	1 gm
Sweetener (sodium saccharin)	0.4 gm
Flavor oils (peppermint, eucalyptus and clove oils)	1.5 ml

Polyoxyethylene (20) sorbitan monostearate	3 gm
Ethanol	100 ml
Sorbitol solution	200 gm
Purified water (qs)	1000 ml

Method of dispensing: Dissolve cetylpyridinium chloride, citric acid and sodium saccharin in a sufficient amount of the water and add ethanol. Mix polyoxyethylene (20) sorbitan monostearate and flovor oils and add slowly hydroalcoholic solution with stirring, sorbitol and mix. Add sufficient amount of purified water to produce 1000 ml.

GARGLES

Gargles are aqueous and hydroalcoholic solution which is used to treat or prevent throat infection. They are dispensed in concentrated form with directions for dilution with warm water. They are brought into intimate contact with the mucous membrane of the throat and allow to remain for a few moments. They are used for deodorizing and antibacterial effect.

They are usually available in concentrated form with direction for dilution with warm water before use. They are brought into intimate contact with the mucous membrane of the throat and are allowed to remain in contact with it for a few seconds, before they are thrown out of the mouth, they are used to relieve soreness in mild throat infection. It also stimulates secretion of saliva which relieves dryness, e.g. phenol gargles, potassium chloride and phenol gargles.

Storage: Store at room temperature keep out of the reach of children. Store away from direct sunlight, heat and moisture.

Labeling: The containers should be labeled "For external use only". The direction for proper dilution should be stated on the label.

Example: Prepare and dispense 100 ml of potassium chlorate and phenol gargle BPC.

Potassium chlorate and phenol gargles BPC.

Potassium chlorate	30.0 gm
Patent blue V	0.009 gm
Liquefied phenol	15.0 ml
Water sufficient to make	1000 ml

Method: Dissolve the potassium chlorate in warm water. Cool and add liquefied phenol. Add the dye solution, filter and make up volume. Transfer to a container, cork, label and dispense.

LINIMENTS

Liniments are solution or mixture of various substances in oil, alcoholic solution of soap or emulsions or occasionally semi-solid preparations intended for external application and should by labeled "For external use only". They are applied with rubbing or massaged into the skin as counterirritating or stimulating agents to the affected area.

Liniments are usually applied with friction and rubbing of the skin. The oil or soap base proving base of application and message. Alcoholic liniments are used generally for their rubifacient, counterirritant, mildly astringents and show penetrating effects. These types of liniments easily penetrate to the skin.

The oily liniments are slow in their action but are more useful when massaged. The function of liniment depends on the additives but most of liniments may function solely as protective coating on the affected area. Liniment should not be applied to the broken skin because they would be very irritating especially if alcohol is used as solvent.

They may Contain Following Substances

a. Analgesic
b. Antimicrobial
c. Rubifacient
d. Counterirritant
e. Stimulants
f. Soothing agents.

Although alcohol is primarily used as solvent, it enhances the penetration of the medicaments into the skin and has counterirritant or rubifacient action. Counter irritants are used to mask pain from fibrositis, sciatica, neuralgia and similar complaints by producing warmth, tingling and numbness. When rubbed onto the skin, they also cause redness and hence are called rubifacient. Cotton oil and arachis oil are less irritant than alcohol and spread more easily on the skin.

Two types of vehicle are used for the preparation of liniments (i) alchol, e.g. soap liniments and aconite liniments, and (ii) oils, e.g. camphor liniment and methyl salicylate liniment.

Labeling

It should be comply with the general requirements for labeling. In addition, the labeling on the container should indicate—for external use only, shake well before use, not to be applied to wounds or broken skin, store in cool place.

Container

Narrow mouthed screw-capped bottles can be used for dispensing liniments.

Example: *Prepare and dispense white liniment.*

R_x	
Oleic acid	85 ml
Turpentine oil	250 ml
Dilute ammonia solution	45 ml
Ammonium chloride	125 gm
Purified water	1000 ml

Method of dispensing: Mix the oleic acid with measured quantity of turpentine oil. Mix dilute ammonia solution with 45 ml of purified water and warm it. Add warm diluted ammonia solution to the oily solution and shake to form an emulsion. Finally make up the volume with purified water.

Example: *Prepare and dispense camphor liniment.*

R_x	
Camphor	200 gm
Arachis oil	800 gm (qs)

Method of dispensing: Mix weighted amount of camphor in arachis oil in a closed vessel. Finally make up the volume with arachis oil.

Example: Prepare and dispense soap liniment.

R_x	
Soft soap	10 gm
Capmhor	10 gm
Lemon grass oil	40 gm
Purified water	15 ml
Alcohol (90.0%)	170 ml (qs)

Method of dispensing: Dissolve the weighted quantity of soap, camphor and lemon grass oil in alcohol. Add purified water and remaining amount of alcohol to make up the volume and mix.

Keep aside for a week and filter to remove the undissolved substance.

Example: Prepare and dispense turpentine liniment.

R_x	
Soft soap	50 gm
Camphor	50 gm
Turpentine oil	650 gm
Purified water	1000 gm (qs)

Method of dispensing: Mix the soft soap with small amount of purified water (100 ml). Make solution of camphor in fresh rectified turpentine oil. Gradually add camphor solution to the soap mixture with trituration until a thick creamy emulsion is formed. Finally add sufficient amount of purified water to make the volume and mix.

Example: Prepare and dispense calamine liniment.

R_x	
Calamine	50 gm
Wool fat	10 gm
Oleic acid	5 ml
Arachis oil	500 ml
Calcium hydroxide solution	1000 ml (qs)

Method of dispensing: Melt weighted amount of wool fat, oleic acid and arachis oil. Triturate calamine with melted oil.

Add calcium hydroxide solution and shake it, transfer it to a suitable container and shake vigorously and finally make up the volume with calcium hydroxide solution.

INHALATION

Inhalants are a broad range of drugs in the forms of gases, aerosols, or solvents which are breathed in and absorbed through the lungs. While some inhalant drugs are used for medical purposes, as in the case of nitrous oxide (a dental anesthetic) a small number of recreational inhalant drugs are used illicitly, such as anesthetics (ether and nitrous oxide) and volatile anti-angina drugs (alkyl nitrites).

Inhalant users inhale vapors or aerosol propellant gases using plastic bags held over the mouth or by breathing from an open container of solvents, such as gasoline. Nitrous oxide gases from whipped cream aerosol cans and aerosol hairspray or non-stick frying spray are sprayed into plastic bags. Once these solvents or gases are inhaled, the extensive capillary surface of the lungs rapidly absorb the solvent or gas, and blood levels peak rapidly. The intoxication effects occur so quickly that the effects of inhalation can resemble the intensity of effects produced by intravenous injection of other psychoactive drugs.

Working of Inhalant

Shake the inhaler well immediately before each use, then remove the cap from the mouthpiece; and save for recapping canister after each use. If the cap is lost, the inhaler mouthpiece should be inspected for the presence of foreign objects before each use. Make sure the canister is fully and firmly inserted into the actuator.

1. Breathe out fully through the mouth, expelling as much air from your lungs as possible, place the mouthpiece fully into the mouth, holding the inhaler in its upright position (see Fig. 10.1) and closing the lips around it.
2. While breathing in deeply and slowly through the mouth, fully depress the top of the metal canister with your index finger as shown in Fig. 10.2.
3. Hold your breath as long as possible. Before breathing out, remove the inhaler from your mouth and release your finger from the canister.

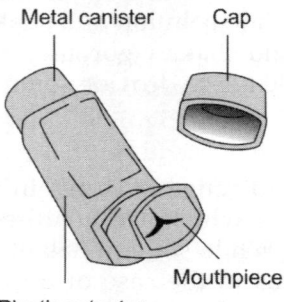

Metal canister   Cap

Mouthpiece

Plastic actuator

Fig. 10.1: Inhaler

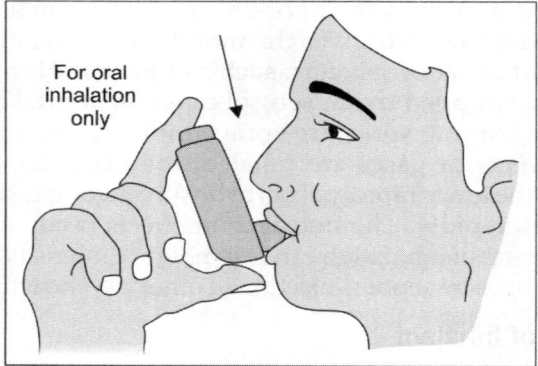

For oral
inhalation
only

Fig. 10.2: How to use inhaler

4. Wait one minute and shake the inhaler again. Repeat steps 2 through 4 for each inhalation prescribed by your doctor.

5. Cleanse the inhaler thoroughly and frequently. Remove the metal canister and cleanse the plastic case and cap by rinsing thoroughly in warm, running water at least once a day. After thoroughly drying the plastic case and cap, gently replace the canister into the case with a twisting motion and put the cap back onto the mouthpiece.

6. As with all aerosol medications, it is recommended to "test spray" the inhaler. Do this by spraying 4 times into the air before using for the first time and when the inhaler has not been used for a prolonged period of time (i.e. more than 4 weeks).

7. Discard the canister after you have used the labeled number of inhalations. The correct amount of medication in each inhalation cannot be assured after 200 actuations from the 17 gm canister, even though the canister is not completely empty. The canister should be discarded when the labeled number of actuations has been used. Before you reach the specific number of actuations, you should consult your doctor to determine whether a refill is needed.

Precautions

- Contents under pressure: Do not puncture.
- Do not use or store near heat or open flame.
- Exposure to temperatures above 120°F may cause bursting, never throw container into fire or incinerator.
- Keep out of reach of children, avoid spraying in eyes.
- Store between 15° and 30°C (59 and 86°F), as with most inhaled medications in aerosol canisters, the therapeutic effect of this medication may decrease when the canister is cold; for best results, the canister should be at room temperature before use.
- Shake well before using.

Example: *Prepare and dispense aqueous inhalation.*

R_x	
Eucalyptus oil	60 ml
Menthol	30 gm
Light magnesium carbonate	65 gm
Purified water	1000 ml (qs)

Method of dispensing: Powder weighed amount of menthol in glass mortar and pestle, add eucalyptus oil and stir unit the solid has dissolved and add other additives and mix well. Finally make up the volume with purified water.

Example: *Prepare and dispense benzoin inhalation.*

R_x	
Benzoin	100 gm
Prepared storax	68.5 gm
Specially denatured spirit	1000 ml (qs)

Method of dispensing: Benzoin and prepared storax should be macerated with 7.5 ml of specially denatured spirit for twenty four hours. Filter and specially denatured spirit passed through to produce 1000 ml.

Example: Prepare and dispense menthol inhalation.

R_x	
Menthol	10 gm
Specially denatured spirit	500 ml (qs)

Method of dispensing: Mix menthol with specially denatured spirit in motor and pestle. Add sufficient specially denatured spirit through filter and poduce 500 ml.

SEMI-SOLID DOSAGE FORMS
Mucilages

Mucilage is a polar glycoprotein an exopolysaccharide a polymer produced by most plants and some microorganisms. The official mucilages are thick, viscid, adhesive liquids, produced by dispersing gum in water, or by extracting the mucilaginous principles from vegetable substances with water. The mucilages are prone to decomposition, showing appreciable decrease in viscosity on storage; they should never be prepared in quantities larger than can be used immediately, unless a preservative is added. Acacia mucilage NFXII contains benzoic acid and tragacanth mucilage BPC (1973) contains alcohol and chloroform water.

Acacia mucilage may be prepared by placing 350 gm of acacia in a graduated bottle, washing the drug with cold purified water, allowing it to drain, and adding enough warm purified water, in which 2 gm of benzoic acid has been dissolved, to make the product measure 1000 ml. The bottle then is stoppered, placed on its side, rotated occasionally and the product strained when the acacia has dissolved and labeled it.

Tragacanth mucilage BPC (1973) is prepared by mixing 12.5 gm of tragacanth with 25 ml alcohol (90%) in a bottle and then quickly adding sufficient chloroform water to 1000 ml and shaking vigorously. The alcohol used to disperse the gum to prevent agglomeration on addition of water (Flow chart 10.3).

Flow chart 10.3: Showing various semi-solid dosage form

Mucilages are used primarily to aid in suspending insoluble substance in liquids, their colloidal character and viscosity helps prevent immediate sedimentation.

Examples: Including sulfur in lotions, resin in mixtures, and oils in emulsions. Both tragacanth and acacia either are partially or completely insoluble in alcohol.

Tragacanth is precipitated from solution by alcohol, but acacia, on the other hand is soluble in diluted alcoholic solutions. A 60% solution of acacia may be prepared with 20% alcohol, and a 4% solution of acacia may be prepared even with 50% alcohol. The viscosity of tragacanth mucilage is reduced by acid, alkalis or sodium chloride, particularly if the mucilage is heated. If shows maximum viscosity at pH 5.

Recent research on mucilages includes the preparation of mucilage from plantain and the identification of its sugars, the preparation and suspending properties of cocoagum, the preparation of glycerin ointments using flex seed mucilage, and the consideration of various gums and mucilage obtained from several Indian plants for pharmaceutical purposes.

Several synthetic mucilage-like substances such as polyvinyl alcohol, methylcellulose, carboxymethylcellulose and related substances are used at the appropriate concentration as mucilage substitutes and emulsifying and suspending agents. Methylcellulose is used widely as a bulk laxative because it absorbs water and swell to a hydrogel in the intestine, in much the same manner as psyllium or karaya gum. Methylcellulose oral solution UPS is a flavored solution of the agent. It may be prepared by adding slowly the methylcellulose to about one-third the amount of boiling waters, with stirring, until it is thoroughly wetted. Cold water then should be added and the wetted material allowed to dissolve while stirring. The viscosity of the solution will depend upon the concentration and the specifications of the methylcellulose. The synthetic gums are nonglycogenetic and may be used in the preparation of diabetic syrups. Sodium carboxymethylcellulose 0.25 to 1% of a medium grade in water is generally suitable for preparing a suspending vehicle. Several formulas for such syrups, based on sodium carboxymethylcellulose, have been proposed, uniformly smooth mucilages sometimes are difficult to prepare because of the uneven wetting of the gums. In general, it is best to use fine gum particles and disperse them with good agitation in a little 95% alcohol or in cold water (except for methylcellulose). The appropriate amount of water then are be added with constant stirring.

CREAMS

Creams are semi-solid dosage forms containing one or more drug substances dissolved or dispersed in a suitable base. This term has traditionally been applied to semisolids that possess a relatively fluid consistency formulated as either water-in-oil (e.g. cold cream) or oil-in-water (e.g. fluocinolone acetonide cream) emulsions. However, more recently the term has been restricted to products consisting of oil-in-water emulsions or aqueous microcrystalline dispersions of long-chain fatty acids or alcohols that are water washable and more cosmetically and esthetically acceptable. Creams can be used for administering drugs via the vaginal route (e.g. triple sulfa vaginal cream).

Pharmaceutical preparations for treatment of conditions such as rashes, skin irritation, stings, fungal infections, etc. are normally supplied in the form of a cream or ointment as this provides an effective means of delivering the active ingredient directly to the required area. Active ingredients are dispersed in either phase or added when the emulsion has been formed and allowed to cool. Ingredients, formulation and product viscosity differ widely, however, a typical manufacturing process breaks down into four individual operations:

- **Preparation of the oil phase:** Flake/powder ingredients, sometimes dry blended in advance, are dispersed into mineral oil or silicone oil. Heating may be required to melt some ingredients.

- **Hydration of aqueous phase ingredients:** Emulsifiers, thickeners and stabilizers are dispersed into water in a separate vessel. Heating may be required to accelerate hydration.

- **Forming the emulsion:** The two phases are blended under vigorous agitation to form the emulsion.

- **Dispersion of the active ingredient:** The active ingredient often makes up only a small proportion of the formulation;

this must be efficiently dispersed to maximize yield and product effectiveness.

Types of Cream

Creams are mainly of two types

1. **Oil-in-water (o/w):** Composed of small droplets of oil dispersed in a continuous phase—o/w creams are more comfortable and cosmetically acceptable as they are less greasy and more easily washed off using water.

2. **Water-in-oil (w/o):** Composed of small droplets of water dispersed in a continuous oily phase. W/o are also more moisturizing as they provide an oily barrier which reduces water loss from the stratum corneum, the outermost layer of the skin. According to the functions the creams can be classified as—cleansing and cold creams foundation and vanishing creams night and massage creams H and body creams all-purpose and general creams.

A. Cleansing Creams

It helps in keeping the body clean and most important and primitive need on account of personal hygiene and beautification which leads to the need of cosmetics. They are used for removal of facial make-up, surface grime, oil, and water and oil soluble soil efficiently, mainly from the face and throat.

B. Vanishing and Foundation Creams

They spread easily and seem to disappear rapidly when rubbed. These creams are composed of emollient esters which leave a little apparent film on the skin. After application the cream leaves a dry but tacky residual film which also has a drying effect on the skin. These are used in hot climates which cause perspiration on the face.

C. Foundation Creams

Foundation creams provide base make-up to hold the powder or other make-up above it. It vary in viscosity and available in the form of liquid to thicker creams. The liquid foundation make-up is much easier to apply than powder and a smooth appearance can be obtained. Night and massage creams are used to provide nourishment to the skin. To supplement foods for the skin and to treat the dry skin nutritive. Creams which are generally applied on skin and left for a few or several hours mostly overnight, known as night creams. Creams which act by providing emollient action by rubbing the cream on the skin with massage like action are called massage creams.

D. Hand and Body Creams

Hand and body creams are used for hands and other body part's skin may be exposed to water, water soap, detergents causes removal of lipids and other secretions from the skin. Cold and dry winds take out moisture resulting in chapping of the skin. Skin dry, scaly, infection due to microbes can leads to dermatitis. So to control all these hand and body creams are applied. The main functions of hand and body creams are to provide an oily film to protect the skin. Keep the skin smooth but not greasy, easy to apply.

E. All-Purpose Creams

The all-purpose creams are also known as 'Sports cream' as they were used by sportsmen in skiing and outdoor activities. They are somewhat oily but not greasy type and can spread easily on the skin to give protective film the composition of these cream is such that it can act—as a foundation cream to provide a foundation base for make-up. As a cleansing cream and liquefy easily. As a cream to smooth the rough surface of the skin. Hence, they are called all-purpose creams.

LOTIONS

Lotions are usually liquid or liquid suspension or semi-solid preparations containing one or more medicaments, intended to be applied to the uniform skin without friction. They are lightly applied on the skin or applied on a suitable dressing and covered with waterproof substance like glycerin to reduce evaporation. They may be prepared by triturating the ingredients to a smooth paste and then gradually adding the remaining liquid phase. For large quantity preparation, high speed mixers or homogenizer are used. A wide variety of ingredients are employed in the preparation to produce better dispersions that show good cooling, soothing, drying or protective nature of the lotion. Following substances are used in the preparation of lotions.

1. **Bentonite:** As a suspending agent.

2. **Methylcellulose (MC) or sodium carboxymethylcellulose (sodium CMC):** To hold the active ingredient in contact with the affected site.

3. **Glycerin:** Keep the skin moist for considerable period of time and to prevent the loss of moisture.

4. **Alcohol:** Used for increased the action like drying, cooling, etc.

5. **Miscellaneous:** Benzocaine, calamine, steroids, zinc oxide, etc.

Lotions are generally prescribed for the following purpose—anesthetic, antiseptic, astringent, germicide, protective, antihistaminic. Microorganisms may grow in certain lotions if no preservative is added. Care should be taken to avoid contamination during the preparation of lotion, even if it contains preservative.

Dilution of lotions: Care should be taken in dilution, particularly to prevent microbial contamination. The appropriate diluent should be used and heating should be avoided during mixing. Diluted lotions should be used within four weeks of their preparation.

Examples

Acriflavine lotion	Dichloroxylenol lotion	Salicylic acid lotion
Boric acid lotion	Gentian violet lotion	Thiomersal lotion
Calamine lotion	Oily calamine lotion	Zinc sulphate lotion
Cetrimide lotion	Dichloroxylenol lotion	Potassium permanganate lotion

Example: Prepare and dispense calamine lotion

R_x	
Calamine	150 gm
Zinc oxide	60 gm
Bentonite	30 gm
Sodium citrate	5 ml
Liquefied phenol	5 ml
Glycerin	50 ml
Rose water, sufficient to produce	1000 ml

Method of dispensing: Prepare sodium citrate solution in 700 ml rose water. Triturate calamine, zinc oxide, and bentonite with citrate solution in a mortar and pestle and add other additives and make sufficient volume with rose water.

Example: *Prepare and dispense boric acid lotion.*

R_x	
Chlorinated lime	12.5 gm
Boric acid	12.5 gm
Purified water, sufficient to produce	1000 ml

Method of dispensing: Mix chlorinated lime and boric acid and dissolve in purified water to produce 1000 ml.

Example: *Prepare and dispense gentian violet lotion.*

R_x	
Gentian violet	10 gm
Ethanol (95%)	100 ml
Purified water, sufficient to produce	1000 ml

Method of dispensing: Dissolve gentian violet in ethanol (95%) and add sufficient purified water to produce 1000 ml.

Containers: Narrow mouthed, fluted bottle.

Label: "Stored in a cool and dry place away from sunlight". The label on the container should contain— "Shake well before use" and "For external use only".

PASTES

Paste are the semisolid preparation meant for external application to the skin. They contain large amount of finely powdered solids like starch, zinc oxide, etc. Due to presence of these substances they have viscosity and stiffness and less attractive cosmetically. Since pastes are stiff they do not melt at ordinary temperature thus forming and holding a protective coating over the area they are applied. They smoothened the inflamed and raw surfaces and minimize the damage done by itching conditions like chronic eczema.

Preparation of paste: They are prepared by trituration and fusion methods, trituration method is used when the base is liquid or semi-solid while fusion method is used when the base is semi-solid or solid in nature. Paste can be applied to the affected part with the help of a spatula or they may be spread on any of dressing material and then applied. They are not removed from the site of application for quite a long time, the pastes are not suitable for application to the scalp because they are very difficult to remove from the hair. Bases used for paste are:

1. Hydrocarbon bases
2. Water miscible bases
3. Water soluble bases

1. Hydrocarbon bases: Soft paraffins and liquid paraffins are commonly used bases for the preparation of pastes.

Example: Prepare and dispense 1000 gm of compound zinc paste BPC.

R_x	
Zinc oxide, finely shifted	250 gm
Starch, finely shifted	250 gm
White, soft paraffin	500 gm (qs)
Make a paste	

Direction: Spread the paste on white lint and apply to the affected area.

Method: Melt the white soft paraffin on a water bath. Separately pass the zinc oxide and starch through sieve no. 120. Mix the required weight of powder in a warm mortar. Add small amount of melted base, with continuous trituration until smooth paste is obtained. Add the remaining part of the base mix until cold and uniform paste is obtained.

Example: Prepare and dispense 1000 gm of aluminum paste, compound BPC.

R_x	
Alluminum powder	200 gm
Zinc oxide	400 gm
Liquid paraffin	400 gm (qs)
Make a paste	

Direction: Spread on white lint and apply to the affected area.

Method: Mix aluminum powder and zinc oxide in a mortar. Add liquid paraffin with trituration thoroughly until smooth paste is obtained.

1. **Water miscible bases:** Emulsifying ointment is used as a water miscible base for the preparation of pastes. Similarly glycerin is also used as water miscible base for the preparation of pastes.

Example: Prepare and dispense 500 gm of resorcinol and sulfur paste BPC.

R_x

Resorcinol, finely shifted	25 gm
Precipitated sulfur	25 gm
Zinc oxide, finely shifted	200 gm
Emulsifying ointment	250 gm
Make a paste	

Direction: To be applied on the affected area where dandruff is severe.

Method: Triturate the zinc oxide, the resorcinol and precipitated sulfur with a portion of the emulsifying ointment until smooth and gradually incorporate the remaining part of the emulsifying ointment.

1. **Water soluble bases:** Suitable combination of high and low molecular weight polyethylene glycols is mixed together to get product of desired consistency which soften or melt when applied to the skin. These bases are water soluble. Water soluble dental paste containing neomycin sulfate is prepared with macrogol base.

Method of Preparation of Pastes

Pastes are prepared by trituration and fusion methods just like ointments. The trituration method is used only in those cases where the base is liquid or semi-solid. The fusion method is used when the base is semi-solid or solid in nature. These two methods have already been explained in detail under the topic of preparation of ointments (Table 10.4).

Table 10.4: Differentiation between pastes and ointments

Pastes	Ointments
1 They contain large amount of finely powdered solids such as starch, zinc oxide, calcium carbonate, etc.	1 They contain medicaments which are generally dissolved/ suspended/emulsified in the base
2 They are very thick and stiff	2 They are soft semisolid preparations
3 They are less greasy	3 They are more greasy
4 They are generally applied with a spatula or spread on lint	4 They are simply applied on the skin
5 They form a protective coating to the area where it is applied	5 They are used as protective or emollient for the skin
6 Paste contains a large amount of powder which is porous in nature, hence perspiration can escape	6 They are used for the protection of lesions
7 They are less macerating than ointments	7 They are more macerating in action

Storage of Pastes

The pastes should be stored in a well-closed container and in a cool place so as to prevent evaporation of moisture present in the paste.

PRACTICE QUESTIONS
Very Short Answer Type Questions

1. Why is glycerin used as a base in throat paint?
2. How mouthwash is to be used?
3. Why inhalations are packed underpressure?
4. Enlist the major uses of inhalants.
5. Write the significance of oral dosage from.

Short Answer Type Questions

6. Explain the various adjuncts used in the formulation of mixtures.

7. What are syrups? Differentiate between simple syrup IP and BP.

8. Write the advantages and disadvantages of syrups.

9. Why are the various additives needed in preparing different monophasic liquid dosage form?

10. What are the adavantages and disadvantages of powder dosage from?

11. Classify different types of mixtures.

12. Differentiate between syrup and elixir.

13. Write the difference between lotion and liniment.

Long Answer Type Questions

14. What are mixtures? Classify different types of mixtures. Describe in brief the method of dispensing the mixtures containing:
    a. Indiffusible solids
    b. Precipitate forming liquids.

15. What are syrups? How are they differ from elixirs and solutions? Write in brief the different methods of preparation of syrups.

16. Discuss the general method of dispensing of:
    a. Mixtures containing indiffusible solids
    b. Mixtures containing precipitate forming liquids
    c. Mixtures containing diffusible solids

17. What are mixtures? Classify different types of mixtures. Discuss in brief, the various vehicles and adjuncts used in the formulation of mixtures.

18. Define the following terms:
    a. Syrup   b. Elixirs   c. Liniment
    d. Mouthwash   e. Throat paint   f. Paste
    g. Inhalation   h. Lotion   i. Aromatic water
    j. Solutions   k. Paints   l. Spirits

19. Differentiate between the following:
    a. Syrup and elixir
    b. Throat paint and mouthwash

   c. Liniment and lotion

   d. Paints and paste

   e. Syrup IP and BP

20. Write short notes on:

   a. Liniment   b. Gargles

   c. Elixir   d. Inhalation

   e. Throat paint   f. Paste

   g. Syrup   h. Mixtures

21. Give the method of preparation of the following:

   a. Tolu syrup

   b. Iodine paint compound

   c. Turpentine liniment

   d. Calamine lotion

   e. Compound sodium chloride mouthwash

22. Explain the reasons for the following statements:

   a. Mixtures are not prepared to keep them for long period.

   b. Syrups are not prepared in potable water.

   c. Mouthwashes are to be taken in small doses without any dilution.

   d. Soap is included as one of the ingredient in some of the liniment.

   e. Liniment should not be applied to the broken skin.

   f. Preservatives are not added in syrups.

   g. Inhalation should not be disposed to fire.

   h. Before mixing powders they should be sieved to have uniform particle size.

OBJECTIVE TYPE QUESTIONS
Fill in the Blanks with Suitable Words

23. Simple syrup IP is .... solution of .... in water having sucrose .... concentration.

24. Linctuses should be taken in small .... and swallowed .... in order to have .... and .... effect of medicaments.

25. Angle of repose should be between .... for good flow properties and Carr's index should be ....

26. Effervescent granules contains .... due to which carbon dioxide gas is evolved.

27. Colloid is an example of .... mixture while suspension is an example of .... mixture.

28. Match the items of column I and with appropriate items in column II

Column I	Column II
a. Linctuses	i. Are sweet aromatic preparations
b. Liniments	ii. Are liquid preparation meant for external application without friction
c. Elixirs	iii. Are viscous liquid preparation meant for the relief of cough
d. Lotions	iv. Are viscous liquid preparation used for mouth and throat infection
e. Throat paint	v. Are liquid and semi-liquid preparations meant for application to skin with friction

29. Match the following:
   1. Syrups   a. Topical preparation
   2. Suspension   b. Mouth washes
   3. Lotion   c. Biphasic

30. Match the following:
   1. Propyl paraben   a. Mandl's paint
   2. Iodine   b. Preservative
   3. Chloroform water   c. Suspending agent
   4. Bentonite   d. Aromatic water

ANSWERS

23. Saturated, sucrose, 66.7% w/w
24. Quantity, slowly, maximum, prolonged
25. 20 and 30, 5–20
26. Sodium bicarbonate, citric acid, tartaric acid
27. Homogeneous, heterogeneous
28. a (iii), b (v), c (i), d (ii), e (iv)
29. 1-b, 2-c, 3-a, 4-d
30. 1-b, 2-a, 3-d, 4-c

11

Experiments in General Pharmacy

LABORATORY MANNERS

1. Always enter a laboratory with permission.
2. Keep your belongings and other materials properly in safe area
3. Enter the laboratory wearing a clean apron and carrying other essential required materials.
4. Before starting experiment clean your workplace and keep minimum things with you to avoid congestion.
5. Light burners only with matchstick or lighter and never light with adjacent burner or by any other means.
6. Put off burner by closing gas connection knob and not by blowing by mouth.
7. Keep important belongings in rack or pocket of apron for maximum utilization of workplace.
8. Maintain silence in laboratory and ask your teacher in case of any query.
9. Use dustbin for throwing waste material and not on floors or platform or in sink.
10. Put off electrical fans when gas burners are in use.
11. In case of gas leakage, immediately report to lab-assistant or teacher.
12. During any injury report immediately to your teacher for first-aid help.
13. Clean your working place after completion of experiment.
14. Always wash your hands with detergent or disinfectant and with fresh water after every experiment.

15. Do not carry costly things in laboratory which may be lost or damaged.
16. Before leaving your table—check gas connection, water supply and electricity plug and ensure they are off.

GLASSWARE HANDLING

Different types and makes of glassware are used in laboratory for performing experiments. Mostly glassware of borosilicate glass are preferred because of its clarity and heat and chemical resistance. Silica, boric acid and sodium and aluminum oxide are the components of borosilicate glass.

Washing

1. Before use of any glassware wash them under tap water.
2. Use detergent and scrubber to clean and remove adhesive material.
3. Rinse glassware, before use with materials for which it is to be used.
4. If glassware is new, before use soak it in 1% hydrochloric acid for some time because such glassware are alkaline and may affect the results.
5. If glassware contains unwanted sticky material that is difficult to remove then treat it with nitric acid or chromic acid solution.

Drying

1. After washing keep glassware on stand for draining. Carry out drying at room temperature.
2. Glassware for volumetric procedures should be dried in hot air oven. For faster drying of glassware, it is advisable to dry them by hot air using a hair dryer.
3. Dried glasswares are kept covered to protect from dust and any other contaminants from the atmosphere.

Heating

1. While heating any glassware to not leave it unattended because overheating may cause serious problem.
2. Keep hot glasswares in right place and handle it carefully to avoid burns.

3. Do not keep hot glassware on damp or wet surface.

4. Use pair of tongs or napkin to hold hot glassware.

Glassware Care

1. Do not leave any sticky material in glassware for long periods.

2. Glassware for reuse must be emptied immediately after use.

3. Label all glassware that contains corrosive or any other chemicals to avoid confusion and accidents.

4. Always clean glassware before and after use.

MATERIALS REQUIRED FOR PRACTICAL

Make a separate small bag for practical which should contain the following:

1. Clean apron
2. Practical note book
3. Journal
4. Graph paper sheets
5. Pencil, eraser, ruler, sharpener
6. Permanent marker pen
7. Butter paper
8. Dusting and cleaning cloth
9. Calibrated small and big weight boxes
10. Match box/lighter
11. Self-adhesive labels of different size
12. Colored sketch pens
13. Scientific calculator

JOURNAL WRITING

The practical journal should be of 150 to 200 pages for 20–25 experiments. It should be covered with waterproof brown paper. On the cover of the journal stick label containing information as given below:

Name: .... Semester/Year: ....

Subject: .... Roll No.: ....

Name of Institute: ....

Writing in Index

While writing in the index write experiment number, complete aim or title, page number and date on which experiment performed. To have an attractive index leave one line between two titles and draw over it with a black marker to look attractive.

Writing Experiment

Leaving one page blank after index start writing experiment with fresh page. Journal contains three types of pages, namely blank on left side, ruled on right side and graph page in between. Use these pages as mentioned in the following table.

Details of Journal Writing

If page numbers are not printed, write page number on all pages on both sides in a sequence. While writing headings, use official shortforms only as given in table below and avoid using your own shortcuts for different words. Also do not use the word like sol (solution), temp (temperature), etc. in the text.

Ruled page	Blank page	Graph page
Experiment number	Diagram (if any)	Title of the experiment
Date	Observations	Graph number
Title	Observation table	Scale
Aim	Formula	Graph
Requirements	Calculations	
References		
Theory or principle		
Procedure		
Precaution		
Result		
Conclusion (if any)		

Do not copy from seniors or other journals. Try to write journal on your own by taking help of reference books or your laboratory book, use the term properly mentioned as follows.

No.	Words	Proper	Improper
1.	Date 1 Jan 2007	Date Jan 1, 2007 01.01.2007	Dt. J. 1, 2007 01, J. 2007 1st Jan 2007
2.	Page numbers	01, 02, 03	‹1›, (1), [1], $\boxed{1}$
3.	Experiment number	Experiment no. Experiment no.	Ex. no. Expt. no. Ex. no
4.	Requirements	Requirements	Req.
5.	Procedure	Procedure	Proc., proce., pro.
6.	Serial number	S. no., serial no.	s. no., no.
7.	Observation Table	Observation Table	Ob. Table $Obser^n$. Table
8.	References	References	Ref.
9.	Calculations	Calculations	Cal^n., cals.
10.	Conclusion	Conclusion	Concl., $concl^n$.
11.	Observations	Observations	Obs., obs^n.

Aim: Keeping in mind the objective of experiment—write completely the aim of experiment beginning with word 'To'.

Requirement: Divide requirements of the experiment into two parts, namely chemicals and apparatus. All the solid and liquid chemicals including water must be written under chemicals. Apparatus includes glassware, instruments, equipment and accessories.

References: At least one reference should be written for every experiment. While writing references, refer journals such as Indian drugs, Indian journal of Pharmaceutical Sciences or any other journal of your choice and see how references are written. Once the style of writing (sequence) a reference is selected continue it for all other experiments.

Theory: Under theory part of experiment write definition, classification, principle, formula, method, applications and other related information that can be helpful while studying for *viva voce*.

Procedure: The first important point is to write procedure in past tense because you are narrating the way you have worked for experiments. Avoid style of writing in passage form. It is always better to follow stepwise procedure for better understanding of sequence of work and for representation. Procedure should be brief to understand the way of performing each step.

Observations: Under observations you need to write conditions that were observed while performing a particular experiment.

Observation table: Draw complete observation table giving sufficient column width and row space. If keywords are used in table, meaning of keywords should be mentioned immediately after table. Remember to specify units.

Calculations: You may have to calculate number of parameters. While doing this, give heading for calculation of each parameter. For highlighting the answer, underline it or put it in a square box or brackets. Specify appropriate unit to each value obtained.

Result: Conclude the result in compact and truthful manner. Do not forget to specify the unit for observed or calculated values.

Journal checking: Always get your journal checked at next practical. Avoid presenting journal for checking at the end of term. Before submission, check your journal for different entries and see that it is completed in all respect.

EXAMINATION

In most universities throughout India, annual pattern of examination is followed. However, recently a shift over from annual pattern semester pattern is observed. For an examination of 100 marks (practical) either 70 : 30 or 80 : 20 marking scheme is in existence for university and internal examinations, respectively.

No fixed criterion is laid down for marks distribution but generally it has been observed that the distribution of subject matter in relation with marks is as follows.

1. Synopsis (based on theory and practical)	15–20%
2. Experiment	55–60%
3. *Viva voce*	10–15%

VIVA VOCE QUESTIONS

It is observed that as such there are no specific guidelines for asking questions at the time of examination during *viva voce* session. Any question related to the subject, either from theory or practical or general knowledge, can be asked. Following are a few examples of questions and expected answers.

1. Why are you performing a particular experiment?
   - You should explain the objective of that experiment.
2. How to perform the experiment?
   - Explain stepwise detailed procedure or method of the experiment.
3. What is principle of experiment?
   - Explain principle on which experiment is based.
4. Name other methods of doing same experiment (if any).
   - Give list of other methods.
5. What is the significance or application of the experiment?
   - Explain the application with examples.
6. Different definitions related with experiment.
   - Definition must cover all points so that it can have meaning.
7. Name instrument or equipment used with its parts in the experiment.
   - Answer correct name of instrument or equipment with its parts.
8. Various standard values of properties or parameters can be asked.
   - When standard values are asked, your answer should be with the unit of the same.
9. Any questions from other subjects of pharmacy related with experiment performed may be asked.
   - To answer such type of questions, you have to attend all theory lectures and practicals. Listen to your teachers when they explain. Also make habit of reading reference books and subject related journals.

EXPERIMENT 1

Object: To prepare 100 ml of chloroform water (BP), label and dispense it in a suitable container.

Theory: Aromatic water is also known as medicated water, they are usually dilute saturated aqueous solution of volatile oil or volatile substances. Aromatic waters may be prepared either by diluting the concentrated water or by shaking the volatile substances with water. Some of them have a mild therapeutic action but mainly they are used as flavoring agents in preparation meant for internal administration of drugs. Aromatic waters include chloroform water, camphor water, rose water, cinnamon water, peppermint water and anise water.

Chloroform is easily soluble in water of strength 1 : 200. Hence, there is no need of adding agents such as distributing agent. Chloroform decomposes in presence of oxygen, by these reaction chloroform produce a toxic chemical called phosgene

$$CHCl_3 \xrightarrow[\text{Sunlight}]{[O]} \underset{\text{Phosgene}}{COCl_2} + HCl$$

Store it in amber colored bottle filled up to brim, amber colored prevent photo-oxidation and when completely filled up to brim there will be least chances of aerial oxidation.

Materials: Measuring cylinder, pipette, beaker, amber colored bottle, glass rod.

Reagents: Chloroform, distilled water

Formula

S. No.	Ingredients	Quantity given	Quantity taken
1.	Chloroform	2.5 ml	0.25 ml
2.	Distilled water (qs)	1000 ml	100 ml

Procedure

1. Take a little quantity of water in measuring cylinder.
2. Add required quantity of chloroform.
3. Shake well so that chloroform get mixed with water.
4. Add more amount of water to make up the volume.
5. Transfer it into the bottle and label and dispense it.

Category: Pharmaceutical aid

Storage: Stored in a *"Well-closed air tight container, away from sunlight"*.

Uses

1. As a pharmaceutical aid
2. It has got flavouring, sweetening and preservative action hence it is used in various pharmaceutical formulation for internal use
3. Also used as menstrum for the extraction of crude drugs.
4. As a sedative in cough, asthma.

EXPERIMENT 2

Object: To prepare 100 ml of camphor water (BP), label and dispense it in a suitable container.

Theory: Aromatic water is also known as medicated water, they are usually dilute saturated aqueous solution of volatile oil or volatile substances. Aromatic waters may be prepared either by diluting the concentrated water or by shaking the volatile substances with water. Some of them have a mild therapeutic action but mainly they are used as flavoring agents in preparation meant for internal administration of drugs. Aromatic waters include chloroform water, camphor water, rose water, cinnamon water, peppermint water and anise water.

Camphor is soluble in water in the ratio 1 : 700 camphor is freely soluble in alcohol hence camphor is dissolved in alcohol. Add water till the solution forms a clear transparent preparation Finally add water to make up the volume. Alcohol used acts as a distributing agent.

Materials: Measuring cylinder, beaker, glass rod, mortar and pestle.

Reagents: Camphor, alcohol, distilled water

Formula

S. No.	Ingredients	Quantity given	Quantity taken
1.	Camphor	60 gm	6 gm
2.	Alcohol	600 ml	60 ml
3.	Distilled water (qs)	1000 ml	100 ml

Procedure

1. Take required amount of camphor in a mortar
2. Add to it the required amount of alcohol slowly with constant stirrings so that camphor dissolved in alcohol.
3. Add water to make up the volume.
4. Transfer it into the bottle, label and dispense it.

Category: As a pharmaceutical aid.

Storage: Stored in a *"Well-closed air tight container, away from sunlight".*

Uses

1. As an antiseptic in eye lotion.
2. As a flavoring agent.
3. As an anesthetic.

EXPERIMENT 3

Object: To prepare 100 ml of rose water (BP), label it and dispense it in a suitable container.

Theory: Aromatic water is also known as medicated water, they are usually dilute saturated aqueous solution of volatile oil or volatile substances. Aromatic waters may be prepared either by diluting the concentrated water or by shaking the volatile substances with water. Some of them have a mild therapeutic action but mainly they are used as flavoring agents in preparation meant for internal administration of drugs. Aromatic waters include chloroform water, camphor water, rose water, cinnamon water, peppermint water and anise water.

Rose tincture is a saturated solution of volatile oil. It is insoluble in water hence alcohol is used as a solubilizing agent. Rose water is diluted with an equal volume of distilled water. It is used as a vehicle (solvent).

Materials: Measuring cylinder, pipette and beaker.

Reagents: Rose tincture, alcohol, distilled water.

Formula

S. No.	Ingredients	Quantity given	Quantity taken
1.	Rose tincture	60 ml	6 ml
2.	Alcohol	600 ml	60 ml
3.	Distilled water (qs)	1000 ml	100 ml

Procedure

1. Take required quantity of alcohol in measuring cylinder.
2. Add required amount of rose tincture.
3. Shake well so that rose tincture gets mixed with alcohol.
4. Finally make up the volume with the help of distilled water.
5. Transfer it into a bottle label and dispense it.

Category: As a flavoring agent.

Storage: Stored in a *"Well-closed air tight container, away from sunlight"*.

Uses

1. In perfume industry.
2. Used in lozenges and dentrifices.

EXPERIMENT 4

Object: To prepare 100 gm of simple syrup (IP), label it and dispense it in a suitable container.

Theory: Syrups are concentrated oral solutions of sugar or nearly saturated solutions of sucrose in water or other aqueous liquids. Syrups containing 85% w/v or 66.7% w/w sucrose will retard the growth of microorganisms. Dilute solution of sucrose provides an excellent nutritional media for the growth of yeast, moulds and other microorganisms. When heat is employed for the preparation of syrups, a small portion of sucrose changes to dextrose and levulose. This phenomenon is called inversion. Sucrose solution is optically active and rotates polarized light to right while on heating optical activity decreases rotated the light to left due to formation of other compounds (dextrose ad levulose). The rate of inversion is enhanced by the presence of acids and hydrogen ions, which act as catalyst.

Syrups are Mainly of Three Types

1. **Simple syrup:** It contains sucrose in purified water alone or in combination of other polyols such as glycerin or sorbitol. These substances are added in syrups to reduce the crystallization of sucrose or improve the solubility of excipients.

2. **Medicated syrup:** It contains some added medicinal substances in the syrups and used for therapeutic purpose, e.g. ephedrine sulphate syrup.

3. **Flavored syrup:** It contains various aromatic or pleasantly flavored substances but are non-medicated and generally used as vehicle or as a flavoring agent or for preservation.

Sucrose syrup is a sweet, viscous, concentrated aqueous solution of sucrose or other sugars in water or any other suitable aqueous vehicle. They are used as sweetening and flavoring agents. Examples are lemon syrup, raspberry syrup, tolu syrup, etc.

Syrup is used for the following purpose

1. Syrup retards oxidation.
2. It prevents decomposition of many vegetable substances.
3. They are palatable.

Materials: Measuring cylinder, beaker, and glass rod.

Reagents: Sucrose, distilled water.

Formula

S. No.	Ingredients	Quantity given	Quantity taken
1.	Sucrose	667 gm	66.7 gm
2.	Distilled water (qs)	1000 gm	100 gm

Procedure

1. Take a required quantity of sucrose.
2. Add 3/4th volume of water and stirred till all the sucrose dissolve.
3. Finally add water to make up the required quantity.
4. Label it and dispense it in a suitable container.

Category: Pharmaceutical aid and vehicle.

Storage: *"Stored in a well-closed container, keep in a cool and dry place".*

Uses

1. It is used as a sweetening agent
2. As a vehicle in preparation of liquid dosages form.

EXPERIMENT 5

Object: To prepare 100 ml of chloroform spirit (IP), label and dispense it in a suitable container.

Theory: Spirits are alcoholic or hydroalcoholic preparations containing volatile substances. The volatile ingredient may be in the form of solid, liquid or gas. They are generally used for internal as well as externally as inhalations for their medicinal value while there major use is as flavoring agent. They may be used in the formulation of aromatic waters or as pharmaceutical aids.

Spirits are prepared by following methods

1. Simple solution
2. Solution with maceration
3. Chemical reaction
4. Distillation

Materials: Measuring cylinder, beaker, amber colored bottle, glass rod.

Reagents: Chloroform, alcohol (90%)

Formula

S. No.	Ingredients	Quantity given	Quantity taken
1.	Chloroform	50 ml	5 ml
2.	Acohol 90% (qs)	1000 ml	100 ml

Procedure

1. Take a little quantity of alcohol in measuring cylinder.
2. Add required quantity of chloroform.
3. Shake well so that chloroform get mixed with alcohol.
4. Add more amount of alcohol to make up the volume.
5. Transfer it into the bottle, label and dispense it.

Category: Pharmaceutical aid

Storage: Stored in a *"Well-closed air tight container, away from sunlight"*.

Uses

1. As a pharmaceutical aid
2. As a sweetening agent

3. As a preservative
4. Also used as a main ingredient of carminative mixture.

EXPERIMENT 6

Object: To prepare 100 ml of peppermint spirit (BPC), label and dispense it in a suitable container.

Theory: Spirits are alcoholic or hydroalcoholic preparations containing volatile substances. The volatile ingredient may be in the form of solid, liquid or gas. They are generally used for internal as well as externally as inhalations for their medicinal value while there major use is as flavoring agent. They may be used in the formulation of aromatic waters or as pharmaceutical aids.

Spirits are prepared by following methods
1. Simple solution
2. Solution with maceration
3. Chemical reaction
4. Distillation

Materials: Measuring cylinder, beaker, amber colored bottle, glass rod.

Reagents: Peppermint oil, alcohol (90%)

Formula

S. No.	Ingredients	Quantity given	Quantity taken
1.	Peppermint oil	100 ml	10 ml
2.	Acohol 90% (qs)	1000 ml	100 ml

Procedure

1. Take a little quantity of alcohol in measuring cylinder.
2. Add required quantity of peppermint oil.
3. Shake well so that peppermint get mixed with alcohol.
4. Add more amount of alcohol to make up the volume.
5. Transfer it into the bottle, label and dispense it.

Category: Pharmaceutical aid.

Storage: Stored in a *"well-closed air tight container, away from sunlight"*.

Uses

1. As a pharmaceutical aid
2. As a sweetening agent
3. Also used as a main ingredient of carminative mixture.

EXPERIMENT 7

Object: To prepare 100 ml of calamine lotion (IP), label it and dispense it in a suitable container.

Theory: These are liquid preparation, meant for external application without friction. Lotion may be used for local application such as cooling and soothing and protective purpose. They are generally applied for antiseptic action. Alcohol is sometimes included in aqueous lotion for its cooling and soothing effect. Calamine is a combination of zinc carbonate mixed with ferric oxide, which gives pink color to it. Zinc oxide has got astringent, protective and antiseptic action. Bentonite (colloidal hydrated aluminum silicate) is used for its suspending property. It helps to suspending the insoluble calamine in distilled water. Sodium citrate acts as deflocculating agent or peptizing agent, i.e. prevents the lotion from being too viscous, it also act as a buffer and maintain the pH appropriate to skin. Liquid phenol is an antiseptic as well as preservative. Glycerin acts as an emollient (smoothening effect) and as an humectant (prevents the loss of moisture from the skin).

Material required: Mortar and pastel, beaker, measuring cylinder, glass rod, and bottle.

Reagents: Calamine, zinc oxide, bentonite, sodium citrate, glycerin, liquefied phenol, lavender oil, distilled water.

Formula

S. No.	Ingredients	Quantity given	Quantity taken
1.	Calamine	150 gm	15 gm
2.	Zinc oxide	50 gm	5 gm
3.	Bentonite	30 gm	3 gm
4.	Sodium citrate	5 gm	0.5 gm
5.	Liquid phenol	5 ml	0.5 ml
6.	Glycerin	50 ml	5 ml
7.	Lavender oil	1 ml	0.01
8.	Distilled water (qs)	1000 ml	100 ml

Procedure

1. Weigh the required amount of calamine, zinc oxide and bentonite.
2. Transfer it in a mortar and add a small quantity of water to make a cream.
3. Add required amount of liquid phenol.
4. Dissolve sodium citrate in small quantity of water and mix with above mixture.
5. Add required amount of glycerol and two drops of lavender oil
6. Finally add water to make up the volume.
7. Transfer it to a bottle, label it and dispense it in a suitable container.

   Category: As a protective.

   Storage: *"Stored in a well-closed container, keep it in a cool and dry place".*

Uses

1. It is used to remove roughness of skin.
2. Meant for external application without friction.

EXPERIMENT 8

Object: To prepare 100 ml of methyl salicylate liniment (BP), label and dispense it in a suitable container.

Theory: Liniments are liquid and semi liquid preparations meant for application to the skin. Liniments are usually applied to the skin with friction and rubbing of the skin. The liniments may be alcoholic or oily solutions or emulsions. Alcohol helps in the penetration of medicaments into the skin and also increase its counterirritant or rubifacient action. Arachis oil is used in some liniments, which spread more easily on the skin. Generally liniments contain medicaments possessing analgesic, rubifacient, and smoothing, counter-irritant or stimulating properties. A liniment should not be applied to broken skin because it may cause excessive irritation. Methyl salicylate is water insoluble compound, so we use arachis oil to dissolve it.

Materials: Measuring cylinder, beaker, pipette, glass rod.

Reagents: Methyl salicylate, arachis oil.

Formula

S. No.	Ingredients	Quantity given	Quantity taken
1.	Methyl salicylate	250 ml	25 ml
2.	Arachis oil (qs)	1000 ml	100 ml

Procedure

1. Take a small quantity of arachis oil in a beaker.
2. Add required amount of methyl salicylate.
3. Shaken well so that methyl salicylate gets mixed with arachis oil.
4. Finally add required amount of arachis oil to make up the volume.
5. Transfer it into the bottle, label and dispense it in a suitable container.

Category: Anti-inflammatory agent.

Storage: *"Stored in a well-closed container keep it in a cool and dry place"*.

Uses

1. Used as an analgesic (which relieves in pain)
2. As an anti-inflammatory agent (which reduces inflammation)

EXPERIMENT 9

Object: To prepare 100 ml of turpentine liniment (BP), label it and dispense it in a suitable container.

Theory: Liniments are liquid or semi liquids preparations meant for external application that are intended to be applied to the unbroken skin with friction. They contain substances possessing analgesic, rubifacient, soothing or stimulating properties. Liniments are usually applied to the skin with friction. Liniments should be dispensing in color-fluted bottles in order to distinguish from preparation meant for internal use.

Turpentine oil is the volatile oil and has the action of counter-irritant and rubifacient. This preparation is an emulsion type of liniment, which contains turpentine oil as oil phase and water as aqueous phase. Here soft soap is used as an emulsifying agent to form oil in water type of emulsion.

Materials: Measuring cylinder, beaker, mortar and pestle, glass rod.

Reagents: Soft soap, camphor, turpentine oil, distilled water.

Formula

S. No.	Ingredients	Quantity given	Quantity taken
1.	Soft soap	90 gm	9 gm
2.	Camphor	50 gm	5 gm
3.	Turpentine oil	650 ml	65 ml
4.	Distilled water	1000 ml	100 ml

Procedure

1. Dissolve the soft soap in water and make a smooth solution of camphor in turpentine oil.
2. Gradually add turpentine oil solution to soft soap solution with continuous stirring to form a thick creamy emulsion.
3. Finally add sufficient amount of water to make up the volume.
4. Transfer it into the bottle, label and dispense it.

Category: As a counterirritant and rubefacient.

Storage: *"Store in a well-closed container away from light".*

Uses

1. Used as a counterirritant.
2. Used in myalgia, sprain, and fibrositis.

EXPERIMENT 10

Object: To prepare 100 ml of starch mucilage (IP), label it and dispense it in a suitable container.

Theory: Mucilage is a polar glycoprotein an exopolysaccharide a polymer produced by most plants and some microorganisms. The official mucilages are thick, viscid, adhesive liquids, produced by dispersing gum in water, or by extracting the mucilaginous principles from vegetable substances with water. The mucilages are prone to decomposition, showing appreciable decrease in viscosity on storage; they should never be prepared in quantities larger than can be used immediately, unless a preservative is added.

Materials: Measuring cylinder, beaker, mortar and pestle, glass rod.

Reagents: Starch, distilled water.

Formula

S. No.	Ingredients	Quantity given	Quantity taken
1.	Starch	50 gm	5 gm
2.	Water (qs)	1000 ml	100 ml

Procedure

1. Triturate the starch in mortar with small amount of water to form a smooth paste
2. Add more water and mix well
3. Transfer this suspension to a flask and heat gently with constant agitation
4. The starch becomes gelatinized and forms a mucilage
5. Take the flask from heat and cool it immediately under water
6. Transfer it to a suitable container, label and dispense

Category: Mucilage

Storage: *"Stored in a well-closed container away from light".*

Uses: Used as a emulsifying agent.

EXPERIMENT 11

Object: To prepare 100 ml of kaolin poultice (BP), label it and dispense it in a suitable container.

Theory: Poultice is a soft semi-solid preparation meant for forming an external surface on the body. Poultice contain material, which maintain intimate contact with skin. The primary object of this preparation is to provide tolerable persistent, warmness locally at the site of application. The topical local effect increase blood supply to the area of the application and reduce inflammation.

Materials required: Measuring cylinder, beaker, glass rod.

Reagents required: Heavy kaolin, boric acid, methyl salicylate, thymol, glycerol, peppermint oil.

Formula

S. No.	Ingredients	Quantity given	Quantity taken
1.	Heavy kaolin	527 gm	52.7 gm
2.	Boric acid	45 gm	4.5 gm
3.	Methyl salicylate	2 ml	0.2 ml
4.	Thymol	0.5 gm	0.05 gm
5.	Glycerol	425 ml	42.5 ml
6.	Peppermint oil	0.5 ml	0.05 ml

Procedure

1. Weigh the required amount of heavy kaolin, boric acid, and glycerol.
2. Mix them in a beaker and kept it for 1 hour in water bath.
3. Shake the mixture occasionally and allow it to cool.
4. Separately dissolved thymol in methyl salicylate and added to the mixture.
5. Finally add peppermint oil and mix it well
6. Label it and dispense it in a suitable container.

Category: As a inflammatory agent.

Storage: *"Keep in a cool and dry place".*

Uses

1. For external use as smoothening agent.

EXPERIMENT 12

Object: To prepare 100 ml of benzoin tincture (BPC), label and dispense it in a suitable container.

Theory: Tinctures are alcoholic or hydroalcoholic solution usually containing low concentration of the active principle of vegetable drugs. Tinctures differ from spirits in the sense that tincture contains low concentration of active principles of vegetable drugs while spirits contain volatile substances. When the product contains 45% or more alcohol it is called tincture.

Since tincture contains alcohol hence they are very stable products and can be stored for a long period of time without any preservative.

Tinctures are generally prepared by following extraction methods:

i. Maceration

ii. Percolation.

Benzoin is a resin obtained from Styrax benzoin. It contains benzoic and cinnamic acid esters of alcohol benzoresinol. The finely crushed benzoin offers larger surface area for solvent action and hence facilitate complete and proper extraction of the constituents. Initially approximately 80% of menstruum is used, finally remaining amount of menstruum is added. The preparation is filtered to separate the alcoholic layer from the gummy substance and enough menstruum is passed through the filter to dissolve any adhering liquid from the gummy material.

Materials: Measuring cylinder, beaker, amber colored bottle and glass rod.

Reagents: Benzoin, alcohol (90%).

Formula

S. No.	Ingredients	Quantity given	Quantity taken
1.	Benzoin	100 gm	10 gm
2.	Alcohol 90% (qs)	1000 ml	100 ml

Procedure

1. Take a large quantity of alcohol in a beaker.
2. Macerate the crushed benzoin in alcohol for an hour with constant stirring.
3. Shake well so that benzoin get mixed with alcohol, filter it.
4. Add more amount of alcohol to make up the volume.
5. Transfer it into the bottle, label and dispense it.

Category: Inhalant.

Storage: Stored in a *"Well-closed air tight container, away from sunlight"*.

Uses

1. As a inhalant
2. Mixed with glycerin and water for local application to ulcers, crack nipples and fissures of lips and anus.

EXPERIMENT 13

Object: To prepare 28 gm of ORS powder (IP), label it and dispense it in a suitable container.

Principle: A pharmaceutical powder is a mixture of finely divided drug and or chemicals in dry form. These are solid dosage form of medicament, which are meant for internal and external use. They are available in crystalline or amorphous form. The particle size of powder plays an important role in physical, chemical and biological properties of the dosage forms. There is a relationship between particle size of powder and dissolution, absorption and therapeutic efficacy of drugs.

Powders are classified as

1. Bulk powder for external use
2. Bulk powders for internal use
3. Simple and compound powders
4. Effervescent granules
5. Cachets.

Observation Table

S. No.	Ingredients	Quantity given	Quantity taken
1.	Sodium chloride	12.5 gm	3.5 gm
2.	Potassium chloride	5.35 gm	1.49 gm
3.	Sodium bicarbonate	10.3 gm	2.88 gm
4.	Dextrose (anhydrous)	71.4 gm	19.9 gm

Procedure

1. Weigh the required amount of sodium chloride, potassium chloride, sodium bicarbonate, and dextrose.
2. Mix them in mortar and pestle and pass through the sieve no. –80
3. Dispense the powder and label it.

Category: As an electrolyte replenisher.

Storage: *Stored in a well-closed airtight container, keep it in a cool and dry place.*

Uses

1. Used in dehydration, dysentery and diarrhea.
2. As a electrolyte replenisher.

EXPERIMENT 14

Object: To prepare 100 gm of absorbable dusting powder (USP/NF), label it and dispense it in a suitable container.

Principle: Dusting powder is a fine state of subdivision of such substance for external application. They are usually mixture of substance zinc oxide, starch and boric acid or natural mineral substance such as kaolin or talc, the later may be contaminated with pathogenic organism and should therefore be sterilized by heat. Dusting powders are not intended for oral use. Dusting powder should be passed through sieve number 80 (# 80) before dusting to avoid partial loss. It is better to weigh for some extra quantity, dusting powders are of two types:

1. Medical
2. Surgical

Observation Table

S. No.	Ingredients	Quantity given	Quantity taken
1.	Purified talc	500 gm	50 gm
2.	Starch	250 gm	25 gm
3.	Zinc oxide	50 gm	5 gm
4.	Salicylic acid	200 gm	20 gm

Procedure

1. Weigh the required quantity of starch, talc, zinc oxide and salicylic acid.
2. Mix them in ascending order of their weight.
3. Pass the mix powder through a sieve number 80.
4. After sieving, again mix the contents.
5. Dispense dusting powder in six sub-divided glass, label and dispense it.

Category: As Medical and surgical.

Storage: *"Stored in a cool and dry place".*

Uses: As an antiperspirant.

EXPERIMENT 15

Object: To prepare and submit 20 ml of cresol with soap solution IP (lysol solution).

Principle: Solutions are liquid preparations that contain one or more soluble chemical substances dissolved in liquid solvents. Solutions are generally prepared by four methods:

a. By simple solution.

b. By chemical reactions.

c. By simple solution with sterilization.

d. By extraction.

Solution is a mixture of two compounds, namely solute and solvent. Solute is the smaller component present in the solution and is usually non-volatile in nature. Solvent is the larger component present and is also known as vehicle. Most of the drugs are non-polar or semi-polar. Hence, they cannot be easily solubilized in water. Therefore special methods are used to prepare solutions. Solubility can be enhanced by using co-solvents (examples are glycerin, ethyl alcohol, propylene glycol) or complexation (example is a combination of iodine and potassium iodide) or surfactants (example is cresol with soap solution). Solutions are usually used for their specific therapeutic effect of solute either internally or externally. To increase the shelf life and esthetic value of solutions, various additives are also added such as stabilizers, preservatives, coloring agents, flavoring agents, and sweetening agents. Solutions form most of the dosage forms like mixtures, enemas, mouthwashes, gargles, eardrops, eye drops, etc.

Cresol is a mixture of O, m and p-cresol. It acts as disinfectant. The solubility of cresol in water is only about 3% whereas the quantity of cresol present in this preparation is 50%. To dissolve this much quantity of cresol, a solubilizing agent is required. Vegetable oil contains free fatty acids, which react with potassium hydroxide and form soap. This soap acts as solubilizing agent. The vegetable oil may be cottonseed, linseed, soybean or similar oils, which have a saponification value not greater than 205 and an iodine value, not less than 100. Solubilization is a process which allows a poorly water-soluble solute to go into solution and hence increases the solubility of the materials. It requires the presence of surface-active agents, which form colloidal aggregates when added in higher concentrations. The concentration of the surfactant at which the micelle formation takes place called the critical micelle concentration or CMC. The poorly soluble material either dissolves or gets absorbed onto the micelle at CMC, which ultimately increase the solubility of the material.

Observation Table

S. No.	Ingredients	Quantity given	Quantity taken
1.	Cresol	500 ml	10 ml
2.	Vegetable oil	180 gm	3.6 gm
3.	Potassium hydroxide	42 gm	0.84 gm
4.	Purified water (qs)	1000 ml	20 ml

Procedure: Dissolve the potassium hydroxide in 250 ml of purified water, add the vegetable oil and heat on a water bath, mixing thoroughly, continue to heat until a small portion dissolves in water without separation of oily drops. Add the cresol, mix thoroughly and add sufficient purified water to produce the required volume.

Category: Disinfectant.

Storage: *Stored in cool and dry place, keep away from the children.*

Direction: For external use only as a general disinfectant. It is unsuitable for use on human beings.

Uses: Lysol (cresol with soap) solution is a phenolic compound used as a disinfectant. For domestic or hospital use like disinfection of floors, bathrooms, washbasins, organic waste such as sputum, feces, urine, etc.

Precautions

1. Not to be used in the vicinity of infants such as nursery, children wards, etc.
2. Not to be used in places where food is prepared and served.

EXPERIMENT 16

Object: To prepare and submit 20 ml of aqueous iodine solution IP (Lugol's solution).

Principle: Practically the iodine is insoluble in water; its solubility is 1 : 2950. Iodine in presence of potassium iodide is soluble in water due to the formation of polyiodides. Iodine reacts with potassium iodide to form compounds called polyiodides.

$$KI + I_2 \rightarrow KI.I_2 \text{ or } K$$

The higher polyiodides are more soluble than the lower ones. Hence, a rapid solution of the iodine is affected by using the potassium iodide in concerned solution. Iodine is an essential element of our body and its deficiency leads to development of goiter. The minimum daily requirement of an adult is about 100 µg. This preparation is used in the treatment or perpetrated treatment of thyrotoxicosis. It can also be used an antiseptic. Iodine slowly volatilizes at room temperature therefore, the preparation should be stored in a well-closed container.

Observation Table

S. No.	Ingredients	Quantity Given	Quantity taken
1.	Iodine	50 gm	1 gm
2.	Potassium iodide	100 gm	2 gm
3.	Purified water (qs)	1000 ml	20 ml

Procedure: First dissolve the potassium iodide in a little volume of water. Dissolve the iodine in above solution; add sufficient purified water to produce the required volume.

Category: Internally as source of iodine, externally as an antiseptic.

Storage: *Stored in a well-closed container, the container materials of which are resistant to iodine.*

Uses

1. It is used as an antiseptic and disinfectant, for emergency disinfection of drinking water and as a reagent for starch detection in medical tests.

2. It is a source of iodine.
3. It is used as local anti-infective

EXPERIMENT 17

Object: To prepare and submit 20 ml of strong iodine solution IP.

Principle: Strong iodine solution contains 10% w/v of iodine (limits 9.5 to 10.5) and 6.0% w/v of potassium iodide. KI (limits 5.7 to 6.3). Iodine with potassium iodide forms compounds called polyiodides. The higher polyiodides are more soluble than lower ones. Hence, a rapid solution of the iodine is affected by using the potassium iodide in concentrated solution. Alcohol in the preparation is used as a menstruum. Another advantage of alcohol is that it quickly evaporates when the solution is applied over the skin leaving behind the iodine in very fine particle size. Due to this a larger surface area of iodine comes in contact with the body, which results in quicker absorption. It also dissolves cutaneous fat and hastens penetration and absorption and provides some additional antibacterial effect. The preparation is used as a topical antiseptic agent. The preparation cannot be applied to wounds and abrasions because the alcohol in the tincture is very irritating to open tissues. The preparation is stored in a well-closed container because alcohol and iodine are volatile in nature. The iodine stains the skin, clothes and vessels made from porcelain and metal, therefore, it should be stored only in glass containers. The iodine stain can be removed by sodium thiosulfate solution.

Observation Table

S. No.	Ingredients	Quantity given	Quantity taken
1.	Iodine	100 gm	2 gm
2.	Potassium iodide	60 gm	1.2 gm
3.	Purified water	100 ml	2 ml
4.	Alcohol (90%) sufficient to produce	1000 ml	20 ml

Procedure: First dissolve the potassium iodide in a little volume of water. Dissolve the iodine in above solution; add sufficient alcohol 90% to produce the required volume.

Category: Antiseptic

Storage: *Stored in a well-closed container, the materials of which are resistant to iodine.*

Direction: 'For external use only'.

Uses: Strong iodine is used to treat overactive thyroid, iodine deficiency, and to protect the thyroid gland from the effects of radiation from radioactive forms of iodine.

EXPERIMENT 18

Object: To prepare and submit 20 ml of weak iodine solution IP (tincture iodine).

Principle: Weak iodine solution is used internally in hypothyroidism and externally as antiseptic to treat wounds. In this preparation the concentration of iodine required is 20 mg/ml. As this preparation is used internally as well as externally alcohol 50% (absolute alcohol 50 ml + water 50 ml) is used as a vehicle. Iodine is very slightly soluble in water. Its solubility can be increased using potassium iodide. Potassium iodide reacts with iodine to form polyiodides that are more soluble in alcohol 50%

$$KI + nI_2 \rightarrow KI\, I_2 + KI\, 2I_2 + KI\, 3I_2 + \ldots\ldots\ldots + KI\, nI_2$$
$$\text{Polyiodides}$$

Polyiodides are more soluble in water by ion induced dipolar interaction. Alcohol is used in this preparation because of two reasons: (a) When this preparation is applied to the wounds, alcohol precipitates the proteins and forms a protective layer, (b) Alcohol absorbs heat from the body and gets evaporated thereby causing cooling effect. Since iodine (present in iodine solution) reacts with some ingredients of ordinary glass container, iodine resistant container like amber colored container is used to store iodine solutions.

Observation Table

S. No.	Ingredients	Quantity given	Quantity taken
1.	Iodine	20 gm	0.4 gm
2.	Potassium iodide	25 gm	0.5 gm
3.	Alcohol (50%) (qs)	1000 ml	20 ml

Procedure: Dissolve the potassium iodide and iodine in sufficient alcohol 50% to produce the required volume.

Category: Antiseptic, iodine supplement in hypothyroidism.

Storage: *Stored in a well-closed container, the materials of which are resistant to iodine.*

Direction: 'For external use only'

Uses: As a disinfectant.

EXPERIMENT 19

Object: To prepare and submit 100 ml of aluminum hydroxide antacid suspension.

Principle: Suspensions are disperse systems in which finely divided insoluble solid drug particles are dispersed in a suitable liquid vehicle. The solid particles are known as dispersed phase whereas liquid vehicle is known as continuous phase. A good suspension should have the following characteristics.

1. Finely divided solid particles should not settle rapidly and should be readily re-dispersed on gentle shaking of the container, if particles settle.
2. The suspension should be easily removed from the container.
3. The suspended particles should not form hard cake.
4. The suspension should have optimum viscosity, which facilitates the easy removal from the container and easily spread on the body surface.
5. The suspension should be free from gritty particles.

Suspension should be packed in suitable containers. For less viscous preparations use narrow mouthed bottles, and wide mouth bottles for thick preparations.

Based on the nature of the solids present suspensions can be classified as follows:

a. Flocculated suspensions, e.g. tetanus toxoid suspension.
b. Deflocculated suspensions, e.g. procaine penicillin G suspension.

Aluminum hydroxide gel is an antacid suspension. It is also known as aluminum hydroxide suspension or aluminum hydroxide mixture. It is colloidal suspension, hence does not required the use of suspending agent because of the strong affinity that exists between the dispersed phase aluminum hydroxide and water. As a result there is increase in viscosity and aluminum hydroxide gel gets easily dispersed in water.

Aqueous aluminum hydroxide antacid suspension tends to thicken as gel during shelf life. This gelling accelerated during storage under warm conditions (30–40°C). This problem can be circumvented by the addition of sorbitol in concentration from 0.5 to 7% depending on the concentration of aluminum hydroxide in suspension. Aluminum hydroxide has constipating effect; therefore, it is normally combined with magnesium hydroxide, which provides laxative effect in commercial antacid formulations.

The taste of an antacid must be considered for consumers' acceptance. Sorbitol imparts a cool sweet pleasant taste. The parabens are used as preservatives. Peppermint oil as flavoring agent. Alcohol serves as vehicle. Amaranth solution is added to impart color to the preparation.

Observation Table

S. No.	Ingredients	Quantity for 1000 ml	Quantity for 100 ml
1.	Aluminum hydroxide gel dried	360 gm	36 gm
2.	Sorbitol	70 ml	7 ml
3.	Sodium saccharine	0.5 gm	0.05 gm
4.	Methyl paraben	2 gm	0.2 gm
5.	Propyl paraben	0.2 gm	0.02 gm
6.	Peppermint oil	0.05 ml	0.005 ml
7.	Alcohol	10 ml	1 ml
8.	Amaranth solution	qs	qs
9.	Purified water	qs to 1000 ml	qs to 100 ml

Procedure: Dissolve methyl paraben, propyl paraben, sodium saccharine, and peppermint oil in alcohol in clean dry vessel. In another beaker take nearly one half of volume of purified water and add sorbital solution, mix well. To this solution add the alcoholic solution and stir well. Add Aluminum hydroxide in small proportions with continuous stirring. Add amaranth solution and mix. The entire product may be passed through a colloidal mill or homogenizer. Transfer to a measuring cylinder, add sufficient purified water to produce required volume, mix well, transfer to suitable bottle.

Category: Antacid suspension

Storage: *Stored in a cool and dry place, away from sunlight.*

Direction: "Shake well before use".

Use: As antacid in peptic ulcers and hyperchlorhydria.

EXPERIMENT 20

Object: To prepare and submit 20 ml of liquid paraffin emulsion IP.

Principle: Emulsions are defined as disperse systems consisting of two immiscible liquids, one of which is distributed through the other in the form of minute globules, the system being stabilized by adding the third substance, the emulsifying agent. Emulsions are of two types:

1. Oil in water (o/w), in which the oil is dispersed in the water continuous phase. These emulsions are preferred for internal use. In these emulsions gum acacia, tragacanth and soaps of monovalent bases like Na^+, $NH4^+$, K^+ are used as emulsifying agents.

2. Water in oil (w/o), in which the water is dispersed in the oil, the continuous phase. In these emulsions wool fat, resins, beeswax and soaps of divalent bases like ca^{++}, Mg^{++}, Zn^{++} are used as emulsifying agents.

Emulsions are prepared by different methods. They are dry gum method, wet gum method and bottle method.

While preparing the acacia emulsions for extemporaneous use, primary emulsion formula must be used. Based on the nature of the oil different formulas are there.

Nature of oil	Examples	Ratios of ingredients		
		Oil	Water	Acacia gum
Fixed oil	Castor oil	4	2	1
Mineral oil	Liquid paraffin	3	2	1
Volatile oil	Turpentine oil	2	2	1
Oleo gum resin	Male fern extract	1	2	1

Liquid paraffin emulsion is oil in water emulsion, made by the dry gum method, containing 50% v/v of liquid paraffin (limits 45.0–55.0). Liquid paraffin constitutes oil phase and purified water constitutes water phase.

Acacia is used as an emulsifying agent, which forms oil in water type of emulsion. Tragacanth is used as an emulsifying agent as well as viscosity-increasing agent, which stabilize the o/w acacia emulsion. Sodium benzoate is used as the preservative, especially for the oil phase. It prevents the surface growth of the microorganisms when emulsion is packed. High vapour pressure of chloroform allows it to concentrate on the surface of the emulsion and also fill the empty area of the bottle, which will not allow any growth of micro-organisms on the surface of the mixture.

Observation Table

S. No.	Ingredients	Official quantity	Quantity taken
1.	Liquid paraffin	500 ml	10 ml
2.	Indian gum, in powder form	125 gm	2.5 gm
3.	Tragacanth, in powder form	5 gm	0.1 gm
4.	Sodium benzoate	5 gm	0.1 gm
5.	Vanillin	0.5 gm	0.01 gm
6.	Chloroform	2.5 ml	0.05 ml
7.	Glycerin	125 ml	2.5 ml
8.	Purified water, sufficient to produce	1000 ml	20 ml

Procedure: Triturate liquid paraffin and the chloroform with the Indian gum, the tragacanth and vanillin. Add in one quantity 250 ml of purified water and triturate until a creamy emulsion formed. Add the glycerin and the sodium benzoate dissolved in 50 ml of purified water. Add sufficient purified water to produce 1000 ml, mix well.

Category: Laxative.

Storage: *Stored in a well-closed container; protected from light*

Direction: "Shake well before use".

Uses: It is used as laxative in chronic constipation and also used during pregnancy for the emptying of fecal material in body before surgery.

EXPERIMENT 21

Object: To prepare and submit 20 ml of castor oil emulsion.

Principle: Castor oil is a fixed oil and is not miscible with water. To make it miscible a third substance known as emulsifying agent in the ratio of 4 : 2 : 1, i.e. Oil : water : gum will be used for the preparation of primary emulsion. Gum acacia will be used as emulsifying agent because emulsions prepared with gum acacia remain stable for sufficient long time.

Observation Table

S. No.	Ingredients	Official quantity	Quantity taken
1.	Castor oil	8 ml	5.33 ml
2.	Water	30 ml	20 ml

Procedure

By wet gum method

Thoroughly clean and dry a pestle and mortar. Weigh out 2 gm gum acacia and transfer it to the mortar. Measure 4 ml water and triturate it with gum so as to form mucilage. To this add 8 ml castor oil in small quantities at a time with thorough trituration after each addition. Triturate briskly without ceasing until a clicking sound is produced and the product becomes white o nearly white. At this stage the emulsion is known as primary; emulsion. Add about 10 ml more of vehicle in small quantities at a time with constant trituration so as to get a homogeneous product.

Transfer the emulsion to a measure, add more of vehicle to produce the final volume 30 ml, stir thoroughly so as to form a uniform emulsion. Transfer the preparation to a bottle, cork, polish the bottle to remove fingerprints, label and dispense. "Shake well before use".

Category: Purgative.

Storage: *Stored in a well-closed container; protected from light.*

Director: 'Shake well before use'.

Uses: As a purgative for the free evacuation of espeially causing evacuation of the bowels.

Precautions: Because of its prompt action castor oil should not be administered at bedtime, preferably it should be given early in the morning.

EXPERIMENT 22

Object: To prepare and submit 20 ml of cod liver oil emulsion IP.

Principle: Cod liver oil is fixed oil obtained from the fresh liver of the cod fish. This emulsion is given in case of the deficiency of vitamins. A and D as an anti-rachitic. The emulsion should be protected from light to prevent the degradation of vitamin A.

The emulsion is prepared by the dry gum method. Acacia is the emulsifying agent and tragacanth is the emulsion stabilizer. Saccharin sodium is used as the sweetening agent. Benzaldehyde spirit is used as the flavoring agent and chloroform is used as the preservative.

Observation Table

S. No.	Ingredients	Official quantity	Quantity taken
1.	Cod liver oil	500 ml	10 ml
2.	Acacia, in powder form	125 gm	2.5 gm
3.	Tragacanth, in powder form	7.5 gm	0.15 gm
4.	Benzaldehyde spirit	2.5 ml	0.05 ml
5.	Saccharin sodium	1 gm	0.02 gm
6.	Chloroform	2.5 ml	0.05 ml
7.	Purified water (qs)	1000 ml	20 ml

Procedure: Take the cod liver oil in dry mortar and disperse acacia powder and tragacanth powder in it. Add the required volume of water, as for the primary emulsion formula, all at once to the mortar and triturate in one direction only until primary emulsion is formed. Dilute carefully, transfer to a measure, add the saccharin sodium solution, benzaldehyde spirit and chloroform with constant stirring and make up the volume with purified water.

Category: Source of vitamins A and D (anti-rachitic)

Storage: *Stored in a well-closed container in a cool place.*

Direction: "Shake well before use"

Uses: As a nutritional supplement. Since it is obtained from fish oils, it has high levels of the omega-3 fatty acids, EPA and DHA.

Also as a source of vitamin A and vitamin D.

EXPERIMENT 23

Object: To prepare and submit 5 boric acid suppositories.

Principle: Suppositories are conical or ovoid, solid preparations for insertion into the rectum where they melt dissolve or disperse and exert a local or less often, a systemic effect. Their basis is fat, a wax or a glycerol-gelatin jelly. They weigh 1, 2 or occasionally 4 gm. Earlier, small suppositories known, as cones were prescribed for ear infections and long, very narrow forms, called bougies, were used for nasal and urethral infections. There are virtually absolute today. Medicaments are prescribed in suppositories for these reasons.

1. To exert a direct action on the rectum.
2. To promote evacuation of the bowel.
3. To provide a systemic effect.

Systemic treatment by the rectal route is of particular value for:

a. Treating patients who are unconscious, mentally disturbed or unable to tolerate oral medication because of vomiting or pathological conditions of the alimentary tract.

b. Administering drugs, that cause gastric irritation, such as aminophylline.

c. To produce mechanical action on the lower bowel and facilitate evacuation in the treatment of hemorrhoids, anal irritation, constipation, etc.

d. Treating infants.

Suppositories are usually prepared by melting a suitable base, incorporating the prescribed amounts of finely powdered medicament(s) and pouring the mixture into moulds.

Displacement value: The volume of suppository that occupy in a given mould remains same. The weight of a medicated suppository varies when compared to a plain suppository. It is due to the variation of the densities of the medicament and the base. It means the weight of the medicament may not displace the same weight of the base for the same volume. Therefore, an allowance is made for the alteration in the density of the total mass, due to the added medicament. It is calculated by applying displacement value.

Calculation is done for extra quantity to manipulate the loss during preparation. Boric acid is insoluble in cocoa butter. Therefore mixed with a portion of melted cocoa butter on a warm tile. The warm tile prevents the cooling and solidification of the base during mixing only two-thirds of the base is melted, as this prevents overheating of the base and the formation of unsatisfactory suppositories. When cocoa butter is heated above its melting temperature (about 36°C) and chilled to its solidification point (below 15°C), immediately after returning to room temperature this cocoa butter attains a melting point of about 24°C, therefore cocoa butter must not be heated at higher temperature. Cooling the mould dissipates the contain heat and hastens settling of the base. Over filling of the mould is done to prevent hollows and depressions forming at top of the suppository due to contraction of the base.

Observation Table

S. No.	Ingredients	Quantity given	Quantity taken
1.	Boric acid	120 mg	600 mg
2.	Cocoa butter (qs)	1 gm	5 gm

Note: Displacement value of boric acid is 1.5

Procedure: Clean the suppository mould with hot water and detergent. Lubricate the mould with the lubricant fluid and invert the mould in ice. Weigh the cocoa butter and transfer to a china dish. Melt two-thirds of it on a water bath, remove from the water bath and stir well with until all that has melted.

Warm a small tile on a water bath. Place the boric acid on the warmed tile. Pour half of the melted base on the boric acid powder on the tile and mix well to get a smooth dispersion.

Transfer the dispersion to the porcelain dish and stir well to form a homogeneous mixture.

Fill 6 cavities of the mould to overflow. Allow the mass to set. Trim of the excess with a sharp blade. Keep the mould for half an hour on ice. Open the mould and remove the suppositories. Blot off the excess lubricant. Select the 5 best suppositories wrap and dispense in a neatly labeled box.

Category: Local anti-infective.

Storage: *Stored in a cool place.*

Direction: "For rectal use only"

Uses: As an antifungal and antibacterial.

EXPERIMENT 24

Object: To prepare and submit 25 gm of cold cream.

Principle: Cold creams are typically beeswax-borax emulsions. They are so-called as cold cream because on application to skin the evaporation of water leads to cooling effect. When a solution of borax is added to molten beeswax emulsifying agent is formed because of wax acid and borax, i.e. Wax acid is saponified by borax forming Na-soap (i.e. Na-soap of wax acid). This agent is formed at the interface between oil and water, which emulsifies the mineral oil in water. It is because of beeswax, cream is able to contain appreciable amount of water. These are typically white creams of higher-class free from greasiness, which has firm consistency and on application they liquefy and spread easily.

This cream can be either o/w type (or) w/o type depending upon the ratio of water phase. 45% is considered to be the critical level of water phase, cream-containing water less than 45% is w/o type and cream with water phase more than 45% is o/w type of emulsion. Percentage of beeswax used ranges from 5–15% and borax 5–6% of wt of beeswax. Lesser amount of beeswax gives softer cream and higher amount give stiffer cream. Cold cream has got a neutral pH.

Both w/o and o/w emulsion can be obtained by beeswax-borax which depends upon:
- Ratio of oil to water phase.
- Temperature of preparation.

- Amount of beeswax saponified.
- Other ingredient present.

Observation Table

Sl. No.	Ingredients	Quantity given	Quantity taken
1.	Beeswax	80 gm	2 gm
2.	Mineral oil	490 ml	12.25 ml
3.	Soft paraffin	70 gm	1.75 gm
4.	Cetyl alcohol	10 gm	0.25 gm
5.	Borax	4 gm	0.1 gm
6.	Perfume	Adequate	Adequate
7.	Water (qs)	1000 ml	25 ml

Procedure: Take 2.16 gm beeswax, 1.89 gm of soft paraffin, 0.27 gm of cetylalcohol, 13.2 ml mineral oil in a clean dry vessel and heat on water bath to 80°C. Dissolve borax in water in another vessel and heat simultaneously with the oil phase to 70°C. Add the aqueous phase to oil phase slowly with rapid stirring. Continue stirring slowly after the additions of aqueous phase until the cream has cooled to about 50°C. Add the perfume, mix well. Weigh out 25 gm of cream and fill into jar. At the time of filling the cream, it should have cooled to 40–42°C.

Category: Humectants.

Storage: *Stored in a cool and dry place.*

Direction: "For external use only"

Uses: To prevent loss of water for dry skin especially during winter and skin smoothener.

EXPERIMENT 25

Object: To prepare and submit 25 gm of vanishing cream.

Principle: A cream, which spread easily and seems to disappear rapidly when applied on the skin, are termed as vanishing cream. These creams are composed of emollient esters, which have little apparent film on the skin. Low percentage of oil phase is chosen for the above mentioned reasons. Traditional formula of vanishing cream is based on the stearic acid. The acids melt above the body temperature and crystallize in suitable form so as to be immiscible providing a non-greasy film stearic acid to impart attractive appearance to cream.

Stearic acid makes the cream very white and because of this vanishing cream contains partially saponified stearic acid, free stearic acid and water. Cream made with sodium hydroxide is harder than made with potassium hydroxide. Borax also can be used and these creams are white in color, but the product has the tendency to become greasy. Glycerin is used as humectant that attracts moisture and hydrates the stratum corneum. Glycerin also prevents the cream from drying up. Lanolin is used in modern formula as emollient. Tri-ethanolamine stearate is used as emulsifier, which is obtained by reaction between triethanolamine and stearic acid.

Observation Table

Sl. No.	Ingredients	Quantity given	Quantity taken
1.	Stearic acid	200 gm	5 gm
2.	Glycerin	60 ml	1.5 ml
3.	Potassium hydroxide	4 gm	0.1 gm
4.	Triethanolamine	12 ml	0.30 ml
5.	Preservative	0.2 gm	0.005
6.	Perfume	Adequate	Adequate
7.	Water (qs)	1000 ml	25 ml

Procedure: Melt 5.4 gm of stearic acid by heating along with glycerin to about 70°C on a water bath. Dissolve 0.108 gm of KOH in water. Add Triethanolamine, preservative and warm the aqueous solution to 70°C on water bath.

Add the aqueous phase to the oil phase and stir continuously all the time until the cream has formed. When it has cooled to 50°C add the perfume, mix well. Transfer to a clean mortar and triturate well until a cream of pearslescent luster is obtained. Weigh out 25 gm of cream and fill into suitable container.

Category: Cosmetic.

Storage: *Stored in a cool and dry place.*

Direction: "For external use only"

Uses

1. Used as base for free powder and other makeup.
2. Used as emollient.
3. It gives better complexation to skin and also used for oily skin.

EXPERIMENT 26

Object: To prepare and submit 5 gm of tooth powder.

Principle: Tooth powder is the simplest and cheapest form of dentifrices compare to toothpaste. Tooth powder has less solubility problem in formulation because interaction between components is less in absence of water. Oxidizing agent and fluorides retain their effective concentration longer in tooth powder than in toothpaste. It contains abrasive such as precipitated chalk, i.e. calcium carbonate. It is used in small proportion and mixed with larger quantities of other abrasive. It contain dry calcium phosphate which usually provides the toothpaste the pH ranging from 6 to 8.

It also contain detergent like sodium lauryl sulfate which is necessary to reduce interfacial tension between adherent matter and surface of teeth thereby during cleaning, it helps in penetration and removed matter in the foam produced. It also contains sodium per borate that acts as bleaching agent, which is added to improve the whitening action of tooth powder. They are basically oxidizing agents. Artificial sweeteners such as sodium saccharin is used to an extent of 0.05–0.25%. Flavor such as peppermint oil is used which improves the characteristic taste and sensation of freshness in mouth.

Observation Table

Sl. No.	Ingredients	Quantity given	Quantity taken
1.	Precipitated chalk	810 gm	4.05
2.	Tricalcium phosphate	100 gm	0.5
3.	Sodium lauryl sulfate	50 gm	0.25
4.	Sodium per borate	20 gm	0.1
5.	Sodium saccharin	20 gm	0.1
6.	Peppermint oil	Adequate	Adequate

Procedure

All solid ingredients are requiring being in fine powder:

1. Mix the weighed quantity of sodium saccharine and peppermint oil together with small amount of precipitated chalk in mortar until uniform mix is obtained.
2. In another clean mortar mix sodium lauryl sulfate with sodium per borate lightly by trituration.
3. Add flavor solution to this mix and mix by light trituration.
4. Add Tricalcium phosphate.
5. Mix lightly and then gradually incorporate the precipitated chalk. Mix by light trituration until uniform mass is produced.
6. Weigh about 5 gm of tooth powder and fill in container with perforated top.

Category: Dentifrice

Storage: *Stored in a cool and dry place, away from moisture.*

Direction: To be rubbed on teeth

Use: To prevent tooth decay and maintenance of healthy gum.

EXPERIMENT 27

Object: To prepare and submit 20 gm of toothpaste.

Principle: Toothpaste is a dentifrice and its primary function is to remove adherent matter from the tooth surface with minimal damage to it. It is a common domestic cleaning preparation, which is normally prepared by using mild abrasive agent to which surfactants are added. Surfactant aids in the penetration and removal of adherent film and to suspend removed soil matter. The foam produced has physiological effect in making tooth cleansing more pleasurable. Cleaning function achieved in short time and at body temperature.

The basic processes in the manufacturing of toothpaste are:
- Hydration gelling.
- Dispersion of the abrasive in the gel.

Hydration of the gel is normally done by adding a solid gelling agent to glycerin and part of the water under condition of vigorous agitation. The powder addition may be done in variety of steps. It is usual practice to add active ingredient late in the mixing cycle and to add surfactant and flavor last. This is done to avoid excessive foaming and to reduce loss of flavor.

Glycerin and propylene glycol are added as humectant to prevent the toothpaste drying at the tube nozzle. In order to maintain high solid suspension in stable viscous form, adding gum tragacanth increases the viscosity of liquid phase. Sodium saccharin used as sweetener, sodium lauryl sulfate as surfactant, peppermint oil as flavoring agent, precipitated calcium carbonate as abrasive.

Observation Table

S. No.	Ingredients	Quantity given	Quantity taken
1.	Precipitated chalk	400 gm	8 gm
2.	Sodium lauryl sulfate	12 gm	0.24 gm
3.	Glycerin	250 ml	5 ml
4.	Propylene glycol	60 ml	1.2 ml
5.	Sodium saccharin	0.5 gm	0.01 gm
6.	Sodium carboxymethyl cellulose	10 gm	0.2 gm
7.	Chloroform	5 ml	0.1 ml
8.	Propyl paraben	0.2 gm	0.004 gm
9.	Peppermint oil	Adequate	Adequate
10.	Water (qs)	1000 gm	20 gm

Procedure: Dissolve sodium saccharin and propyl paraben in half the quantity of water. Mix glycerin and propylene glycol and add this to sodium saccharin solution. Weigh out required quantity of sodium CMC and place in a clean dry mortar. Add aqueous solution to the gum and triturate rapidly until a uniform dispersion is obtained. Keep aside for 20 minutes to allow binding agent to swell. To the gel produced add precipitated chalk in small amounts and triturate thoroughly after each addition to obtain smooth paste. Add chloroform, peppermint oil and mix well. Dissolve sodium lauryl sulfate in required remaining quantity of water taken in beaker. Add this solution in to the mortar and triturate slowly then fill into the container.

Category: Dentifrice

Storage: *Stored in a cool and dry place, away from moisture.*

Direction: To be rubbed on teeth with the help of toothbrush.

Use: To clean the teeth and deodorize the oral cavity.

EXPERIMENT 28

Object: To prepare and submit 20 ml of potassium chlorate gargles.

Principle: Generally, gargles are used to relieve soreness in mid throat infections and most have a deodorant effect. A bactericide, e.g. phenol or thymol. It is usually present but not in high enough concentration for significant antibacterial activity; however, it may exert a mild anesthetic effect. Potassium chlorate is included in gargles for its weak astringent effect on superficial cells, which helps to remove the tone of a relaxed throat; it also stimulates the flow of saliva, which relives dryness. The best-known gargles are phenol garlic, potassium chlorate and phenol garlic and thymol glycerin compound.

Observation Table

S. No.	Ingredients	Quantity given	Quantity taken
1.	Potassium chlorate	30 gm	0.6 gm
2.	Liquid phenol	15 ml	0.3 gm
3.	Water (qs)	1000 ml	20 ml

Procedure: Dissolve the weighed amount of potassium chlorate is about 15 ml of water. To this add liquefied phenol and add sufficient water to produce the required volume. Transfer to a container, label and dispense. The secondary label "for external use only" must be attached.

Category: Antibacterial.

Storage: *Stored in a cool and dry place, away from children.*

Direction: These gargles should be diluted with ten times its volume of warm water before use.

Uses: These gargles are used at sialogogue and astringent. Potassium chlorate is a sialogogue (which increases the flow of saliva) and astringent (which precipitate the proteins).

EXPERIMENT 29

Object: To prepare and submit 20 ml of antiseptic mouthwash.

Principle: Mouthwashes are aqueous solutions with pleasant taste and odor used to clean deodorize the buccal cavity. They are very refreshing, particularly to bed-ridden patients. Generally they contain antibacterial agents, alcohol, glycerin, sweetening agents and flavoring agents. In this preparation thymol and borax used as antibacterial agents, alcohol as solvent, glycerin as sweetening agent, sodium bicarbonate can dissolve mucous.

Observation Table

S. No.	Ingredients	Prescription quantity	Quantity taken
1.	Thymol	0.3 gm	0.006 gm
2.	Alcohol	35 ml	0.7 ml
3.	Borax	20 gm	0.4 gm
4.	Sodium bicarbonate	10 gm	0.2 gm
5.	Glycerin	80 ml	1.6 ml
6.	Flavor	Adequate	Adequate
7.	Water (qs)	1000 ml	20 ml

Procedure: Dissolve the required quantity of thymol in alcohol. In another beaker dissolve borax and sodium bicarbonate in water and mix the both solutions. Add glycerin and sufficient quantity of flavor mix well. Add the water to produce required volume.

Category: Antibacterial.

Storage: *Stored in a cool and dry place, away from children.*

Direction: 'Dilute with an equal volume of warm water before use'. 'Not to be swallowed in large quantities'.

Uses: To enhance oral hygiene.

Mouthwash has antiseptic and anti-plaque effect it also kills the bacterial which causes plague, gingivitis and bed breath.

EXPERIMENT 30

Object: To prepare and submit 20 g of non-staining iodine ointment BPC.

Principle: Non-staining iodine ointment BPC is used as a counterirritant. The fixed oils and many fats obtained from vegetable and animal sources contain unsaturated constituents. The iodine combines with double bonds of the unsaturated constituents. Hence, free iodine is not available.

$$CH_3 (CH_2)_7 CH = CH - (CH_2)_7 COOH + I_2 \rightarrow$$

$$\underset{\text{Oleic acid}}{} \quad \underset{\text{Di-iodostearic acid}}{CH_3 (CH_2)_7 CHI = CHI (CH_2)_7 COOH}$$

If complete iodine is not combined then the free iodine gives brown color to the product and leaves a stain when applied. In other words, if complete iodine is combined with unsaturated oils and fats, then the final ointment attains greenish black color. It leaves no stain when rubbed onto the skin. Hence, they are known as non-staining iodine ointments. Iodine is easily soluble in unsaturated oils like arachis oil. To enhance the rate of solubilization, powdered form of iodine is preferred. Iodine solution is heated to complete the reaction between iodine and arachis oil. Heating must be done at not more than 50°C, because at high temperatures iodine sublimes.

Methyl salicylate is volatile in nature. To avoid evaporation of methyl salicylate, it is added when the preparation is at lower temperature. Stirring should be done slowly to prevent air entrapment when the preparation starts thickening. Iodine acts as a counterirritant. Methyl salicylate also serves as a counter-irritant and a flavoring agent. Yellow soft paraffin is used as a base. This is a semisolid preparation. Some quantity of preparation will go waste during manufacture of semi-solids. 2 gm extra is calculated to nullify loss during manufacture of 20 gm non-staining iodine ointment, i.e. quantities of ingredients are calculated for 22 gm.

Observation Table

S. No.	Ingredients	Quantity given	Quantity taken
1.	Methyl salicylate	50 ml	1 ml
2.	Iodine	50 gm	1 gm
3.	Arachis oil	150 gm	3 gm
4.	Yellow soft paraffin (qs)	1000 gm	20 gm

Procedure: Depending on the quantity of preparation to be submitted, the working formula is calculated.

1. Iodine is dissolved in arachis oil at room temperature by simple stirring in a beaker.
2. Heat the above solution on water bath at 50°C with occasional stirring until the brown color disappears (or greenish black color appears).
3. Sufficient quantity of yellow soft paraffin is added (previously heated to 40°C), stirred slowly, cooled to solidify.
4. When the above preparation is at semi-liquid consistency, methyl salicylate is added, stirred slowly, allowed for complete solidification.
5. The ointment is transferred to a tightly-closed wide-mouthed container.
6. The container is capped, polished, labeled, and submitted.

Composition: Each gm contains 47.5 to 52.5 mg of iodine.

Category: Counterirritant.

Storage: *Stored in a cool place.*

Directions: For external use only, do not apply on broken skin.

Uses: The deeply penetrating action of ointment provides long-lasting relief from backaches, waist pains, muscle strains, and sprains.

EXPERIMENT 31

Object: To prepare and dispense 10 gm of face powder.

Principle: Face powder is a cosmetic powder applied to the face to set a foundation after application. It can also be reapplied throughout the day to minimize shininess caused by oily skin. There is translucent sheer powder, and there is pigmented powder. Certain types of pigmented facial powders are meant be worn alone with no base foundation. Powder tones the face and gives an even appearance. Besides toning the face, some powders with sunscreen can also reduce skin damage from sunlight and environmental stress. It comes packaged either as a compact or as loose powder. It can be applied with a sponge, brush, or powder puff. Uniform distribution over the face is achieved easier when a loose powder is applied.

Because of the wide variation among human skin tones, there is a corresponding variety of colors of face powder. There are also several types of powder. A common powder used in beauty products is talc (or baby powder), which is absorbent and provides toning to the skin. A good face powder should produce a smooth finish to the facial skin.

Observation Table

S. No.	Ingredients	Quantity given	Quantity taken
1.	Talc	630 gm	6.3 gm
2.	Kaolin	200 gm	2 gm
3.	Calcium carbonate (light)	50 gm	0.5 gm
4.	Zinc oxide	50 gm	0.5 gm
5.	Zinc stearate	50 gm	0.5 gm
6.	Magnesium carbonate	10 gm	0.1 gm
7.	Color	5 gm	0.05 gm
8.	Perfume	5 gm	0.05 gm

Procedure

1. Take talcum powder, kaolin and zinc oxide is ascending order and mix well in mortar vessel.
2. Add calcium carbonate, zinc citrate and magnesium carbonate in mortal and mix well.
3. Finally add one drop of perfume, mix all the constituents well, label it and dispense it in a suitable container.

Category: Cosmetic

Storage: *Stored in well-closed air tight container.*

Direction: For external use only.

Use

1. For beautification purpose.
2. For reducing perspiration.

EXPERIMENT 32

Object: To prepare 100 ml of strong ginger tincture (IP), label and dispense it in a suitable container.

Theory: Tinctures are alcoholic or hydroalcoholic solution usually containing low concentration of the active principle of vegetable drugs. Tinctures differ from spirits in the sense that tincture contains low concentration of active principles of vegetable drugs while spirits contain volatile substances. When the product contains 45% or more alcohol it is called as tincture. Since tincture contains alcohol hence they are very stable products and can be stored for a long period of time without any preservative.

Tinctures are generally prepared by following extraction methods:

i. Maceration
ii. Percolation.

Ginger consist of rhizome of *Zingiber officinale*. Ginger in moderately coarse powder form offer large surface area for solvent extraction, the drug is powdered and before packing in percolator moistened to facilitate swelling otherwise when swelling takes place inside the percolator the packing becomes tight, now sufficient menstrual is poured and kept aside for 24 hours, the marc is pressed after 24 hrs to recover as much as possible menstruum. Finally filtered to remove the cell debris expelled by expression of the marc (Fig. 11.1).

Materials: Measuring cylinder, beaker, amber colored bottle and glass rod.

Reagents: Ginger, alcohol (90%).

Formula

S. No.	Ingredients	Quantity given	Quantity taken
1.	Ginger	500 gm	50 gm
2.	Alcohol 90% (qs)	1000 ml	100 ml

Procedure

1. It is prepared by percolation method, moitened the drug with menstruum and set aside for 5–7 hours.
2. Pack the moistened drug in percolator, add enough menstruum so as to form a layer over the drug and keep it for 24 hours.
3. Collect the percolate in a beaker, continue percolation until three-fourths of volume of the finished product is obtained.

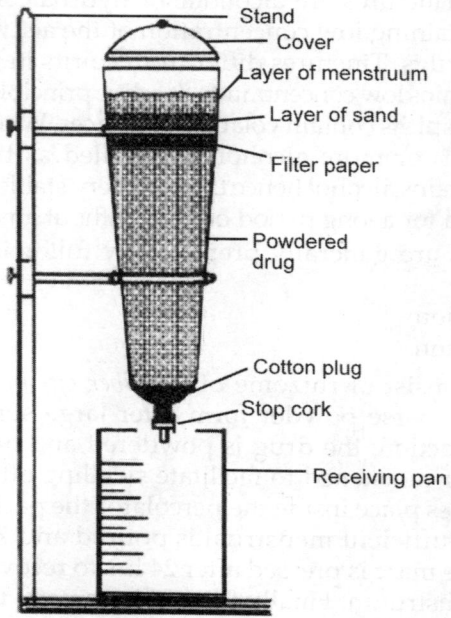

Fig. 11.1: Percolator

4. Press the marc and add more of menstruum to make up the required volume.
5. Allow it to stand, filter it
6. Transfer it to a suitable container, label and dispense it.

Category: Carminative

Storage: Stored in a *"Well-closed air tight container, away from sunlight"*.

Uses

1. As a flavoring agent
2. As a carminative.

EXPERIMENT 33

Object: To prepare 100 ml of liquorice liquid extract (IP), label it and dispense it in a suitable container.

Theory: Extracts are concentrated preparation of vegetable or animal drugs obtained by extracting the active ingredient from the drug using suitable menstruum. They are prepared by maceration or percolation process by using suitable solvent like water, ethanol, and ether as solvent. The extract so obtained is concentrated by evaporation of partial or whole solvent. Finally the residual concentrate or drug is adjusted to formulate it in a suitable formulation.

Unpeeled drug is used because it is more suitable for preparation of extract, a low degree of size reduction is required for the easy penetration of water or other solvents. Chloroform water is added to prevent the fermentation (act as a preservative) of drug constituents. The percolate is boiled for five minutes to coagulate the albuminous matter to remove the viscous material. Alcohol 90% is used to preserve the product. Alcohol prevents the fermentation of product. Fermentation cannot take place in aqueous preparation containing 20% or more of the alcohol. After mixing the alcohol the preparation is kept aside because the substance in the evaporated liquid are water soluble but not necessarily soluble in weak alcohol, hence some precipitation occurs (Fig. 11.2).

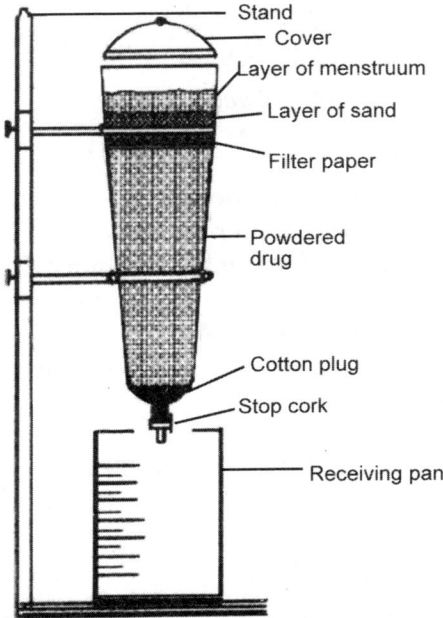

Fig. 11.2: Percolator

Materials required: Beaker, test tube, glass rod, burette.

Reagents required: Liquorice unpeeled, chloroform water, alcohol 90%.

Formula

S. No.	Ingredients	Quantity given	Quantity taken
1.	Liquorice	1000 gm	100 gm
2.	Chloroform water (qs)		
3.	Alcohol (90%) (qs)		

Procedure

1. Percolate the liquorice with chloroform water.
2. Boil the percolate for 5 mins, and set aside for 12 hours.
3. Decant the clear liquid, filter the remainder and mix both the liquid.
4. Evaporate until the wt/ml of the liquid at 20°C is 1.193 gm.
5. After it is cooled and 1/4th of its volume 90% alcohol
6. Allowed to stand for 4 weeks and filter.
7. Dispense the product and label it.

Category: As a mild expectorant.

Storage: *"Keep it in a cool and dry place".*

Uses

1. Used as an expectorant and demulcent.
2. In cough lozenges, cough pastilles.
3. To mask the taste of nauseous and bitter drugs.

EXPERIMENT 34

Object: To study the principle of size reduction using ball mill and to see the effect of:

a. Size of ball, and

b. Number of balls during size reduction.

Principle: The mill works on the principle of impact and attrition.

Theory: Ball mill consists of hollow cylinder mounted on a metallic frame in such a way that it can rotate horizontally on its axis. The cylinder contain balls that occupy 30–50% of the mill volume. The weight of the balls is kept constant. The ball size depends on the size of the feed and the diameter of the mill. The cylinder and balls are made of metal and are usually lined with chrome. In pharmaceutical industry, sometimes the cylinder of ball mill is lined with rubber or porcelain. The balls used in these mills are also made of rubber or porcelain (Fig. 11.3).

Advantages

1. Economical and simple to operate.
2. Large grinding surface within a compact space.

Disadvantages

1. It produces noise.
2. It cannot be used for soft drug.

Materials required: Ball mill, coarse powder, sieves, balance.

Reagents required: Sodium chloride crystal

Procedure: First of all weigh 200 gm of sodium chloride crystal, now these crystals are put into the cylinder of the mill and the mill is rotated. The speed of rotation is very important. At a low speed, the mass of balls will slide or roll over each

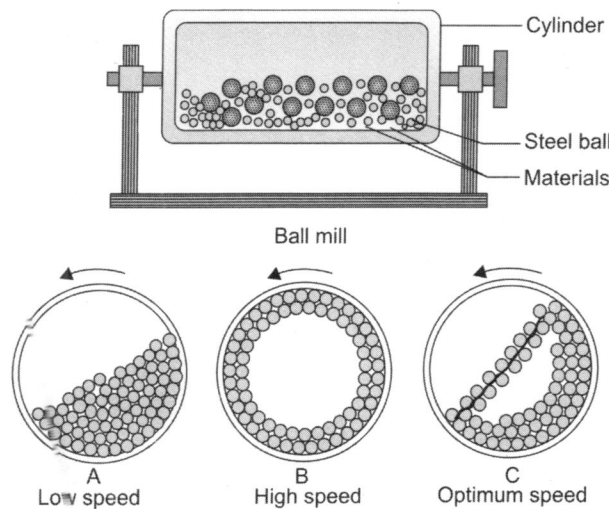

Fig. 11.3: Working of ball mill

other and only a negligible amount of size reduction will occur. At a high speed, the balls will be thrown out to the balls by centrifugal force and no grinding will occur. But at about two-thirds of the speed, the centrifugal force just occurs with result that the balls are carried almost to the top of the mill and then fall in. By this way the maximum size reduction is effected by the impact of particles between the balls and by attrition between the balls. After 30 minutes the material is taken out and passed through a sieve number 40. The amount passing out through sieve number 40 is taken and weighed. Now again repeat the process by taking only small balls, similarly continue the process of size reduction with big balls only. The yield obtained, i.e. the final weight obtained after passing through the 40 sieves are compared and tabulated.

Uses: The mill is used to grind brittle drugs to fine powder.

Glossary

Absorption: The assimilation of one substance by another, where the substance being absorbed diffuses into the absorbing material.

Acid: A chemical compound containing a hydrogen atom that dissociates from a molecule to a hydronium ion in water.

Adsorption: The attachment of one substance onto the surface of another by means of a strong interaction between the two substances or materials. This differs from absorption in that the substances are joined only at the surface.

Aerosol: A dispersion of very small (submicron)-sized liquid droplets or solid particles into a gas. The term is used in packaging as a label for all liquid or semisolid solutions or suspensions dispensed under pressure.

Amorphous: Not crystalline when used with plastics, it means molecules arranged in a random order, without structure.

Ampoule: Glass tubing sealed at both ends, containing a drug intended for injection.

Analgesic: A substance that relieves pain.

ANDA: Abbreviated New Drug Application.

Anesthetic: A drug that stops or suppresses sensations such as pain by affecting either the central nervous system (general anesthetic) or the peripheral nerve structures (local anesthetic).

Angina: A heart disease characterized by intermittent chest pain coupled with feelings of suffocation.

Angstrom: A unit of length equal to one hundred millionth of a centimeter.

Annealing: A controlled temperature method of gradually cooling glass containers in ovens to relieve structural stresses and to make the glass less brittle.

Antibiotics: Substances that inhibit the growth of or destroy microorganisms.

Antihistamines: Substances that neutralize or inhibit the effects of histamine released by the body during allergic reactions or in response to a disease.

Anti-inflammatory: Substances that neutralize or inhibit the inflammation of tissue.

Antimicrobial: Refers to substances that destroy microorganisms.

Antioxidant: A chemical substance that can be added to a plastic resin to minimize or prevent the effects of oxygen attack on the plastic (e.g. yellowing or degradation).

Antipruitic: A substance that relieves itching.

Antiseptic: A substance that inhibits the growth of microorganisms.

Antistatic agent: A chemical substance that can be applied to the surface of a plastic bottle or incorporated in the plastic from which the bottle is made. Its function is to render the surface of the plastic article less susceptible to an accumulation of electrostatic charges, which attract and hold fine dust on the surface of the bottle.

API: Active pharmaceutical ingredient—the active ingredient in a pharmaceutical product.

Aseptic: Free from disease-producing microorganisms. In biologic or medical applications, it refers to an operation performed in a presterilized environment that is controlled to prevent contamination through the introduction of microorganisms. Sterile area that is controlled to remain sterile during operation.

Aseptic filling: The process of combining sterilized pharmaceuticals with sterile packaged in a sterile environment.

Assay: The determination of the concentration of the active ingredient in a pharmaceutical.

Astringent: A substance that contracts tissues or canals, reducing the discharge of fluids.

Autoclave: A vessel capable of containing high-pressure steam that is commonly used to sterilize pharmaceuticals, medical instruments, and medical devices.

Bactericide: A substance that kills bacteria.

Bacteriostat: A substance that is added to a drug formulation to control the growth of bacteria.

Base: A chemical compound that when dissolved in water dissociates to form a hydroxyl ion and raises pH above 7. Generally a metal oxide or hydroxide.

Bioavailability: The availability of an administered drug to the circulatory system.

Blank: The mold parts used in all glass container machines for preliminary formation of glass in preparation for completion of the glass containers in the finish mold where the bottles are blown. The blank forms the parison; hence the parison itself is at times referred to as the blank.

Blister package: A package consisting of a cavity thermoformed from a thermoplastic material and a flat lid stock designed to seal each of the cavities to the edges of the trimmed card.

BTU: British thermal unit.

Buccal cavity: The cavity formed by the cheek.

Buffer: A buffer is a substance that when dissolved in water acts to resist changed in pH that would otherwise be caused by environmental factors (e.g. CO_2 in air or alkaline salts in glass containers).

CAD/CAM: Computer-assisted design/computer-assisted manufacturing (or in printing computer-assisted makeup).

Caplet: A tablet-shaped capsule.

Capsule: A transparent or colored gelatin material, hard- or soft-shelled that contains a drug preparation.

Catalyst: A chemical compound that accelerates the rate of a chemical reaction without being consumed in the process.

CGMP: Current Good Manufacturing Practice (as written and used outside the FDA).

Coefficient of thermal expansion: A dimensionless number that expresses the degree to which a material will expand when subjected to a known and specified increase in temperature.

Copolymer: A polymer made from at least two different comonomers.

Cosmetic: Formulate products used to decorate, adorn, or beautify but which have no therapeutic effect or purpose.

Cream. A medicated preparation based on an emulsion of oil in water.

Deliquescence: Refers to a substance that readily absorbs moisture. Becoming damp or liquid by absorption of water from the atmosphere and then dissolving in the water taken up. This property is found in salts (e.g. $CaCl_2$).

Demulcent: A substance formulated to soothe the part of the body to which it is applied.

Densitometer: For printing, a reflection densitometer is used to measure and control the density of color inks on a substrate.

Density: Weight per unit of volume of a substance.

Depyrogenation: The elimination of pyrogens by heat or chemical processes.

Dermatological: Pertaining to the skin or diseases of the skin.

Die: Any tool or arrangement of tools designed to cut, shape, or otherwise form materials to a desired configuration.

Distillation: The process in which a liquid is purified by transforming it into a vapor, separating the vapor from the impure liquid and then condensing and collecting it.

Diuretic: A drug formulation that increases urinary discharge.

DMF: Drug Master File, a blinded repository for proprietary information that permits the FDA to review the safety and adequacy of a component.

Dosage form: The form of a drug preparation that determines how the drug is administered (e.g. tablet, oral liquid, suppository, parenteral liquid).

Effervescent: Refers to substances that produce a gas, usually CO_2, upon mixing with water.

Efflorescent: Refers to substances that lose water on exposure to air.

EFPIA: European Federation of Pharmaceutical Industries and Associations.

EHIBCC: Health Industry Business Communication Council (HIBCC) and its affiliate International Organization, the European Health Industry Business Communications Council.

Elastomer: A polymer with the elastic characteristics similar to rubber: the ability to best retched at least twice its original length without sustaining permanent deformation.

Elixirs: Syrups containing 20 to 25% alcohol.

EMEA: The European Agency for the Evaluation of Medicinal Products.

Emollients: Substances that soften and relax the tissues when applied locally.

Emulsion: A liquid consisting of a discontinuous, immiscible liquid phase dispersed in a continuous liquid phase.

Enteric: Refers to coatings that delay dissolution until a solid dosage form reaches the intestine.

FD and C: Food, Drug, and Cosmetic Act.

FDA: United States Food and Drug Administration.

FFDCA: Federal Food, Drug, and Cosmetic Act.

Filtration: The process by which solid particles are removed from a liquid by passing the liquid through a porous medium whose pores are so small that the solid particles will not pass through them.

Flint: A term used to describe a glass color that is perfectly clear and transparent.

Fluidized bed: A group of solid particles in a container that are agitated by the upward flowing stream of gas. The particles appear as a cloud in the bottom of the confining space.

Fluorocarbon: An organic compound containing fluorine.

Flux: A substance or mixture used to promote the fusion of metals or minerals. Can be called a fluxing agent.

Free radical: A highly reactive species formed by the rupture of a chemical bond.

Gastrointestinal: The system of body organs that included the stomach and small intestine.

Gel: A colloidal semisolid consisting of a networked structure of suspended, fine, solid particles surrounded by a liquid. Differs from a colloidal solution, which has no solid particles to confer some rigidity to the structure.

Gelatin: A water soluble substance extracted from animal tissue and bones and used in the manufacturing of capsules.

Generic: Used in the pharmaceutical business to describe any drug that is labeled for sale with its technical name rather than a trade name, and usually manufactured by companies that were not the original developer of the product.

Glass: The USP on the basis of performance in chemical durability tests specifies four types of glass. Types 1, 2, and 3 are intended for packaging parenteral preparations and type NP for nonparenteral products.

HDPE: High-density polyethylene.

Head space: The space between the level of the contents of a container and the closure of the container.

Hermetic seal: Any seal or any container so sealed that is impervious to all gasses under normal conditions of handling and storage.

HIBCC: Health Industry Business Communication Council and its affiliate international organization, the European Health Industry Business Communications Council (EHIBCC).

Hologram: The image formed by a lensless photographic process (holography) that uses laser light to produce three-dimensional images.

Hormone: A substance formed in and secreted by the endocrine glands. May be made synthetically.

Hydrocarbon: An organic compound containing only carbon and hydrogen.

Hydrolysis: Reaction of a compound with water, resulting in destruction of the compound and the formation of at least two new ones.

Hypertonic: Having a greater osmotic pressure than blood plasma, lacrimal fluid, or interstitial fluid. It can be applied more specifically to a fluid in which cells shrink.

Hypoglycemia: An abnormally small concentration of glucose in the circulating blood.

In vitro: Refers to chemical or physical tests of drugs using laboratory procedures and apparatus (in glass).

In vivo: Refers to tests of drugs in laboratory tissue, animals, and humans (in life).

IND: Investigational New Drug.

Induction heating: Heating a metal object by application of an external magnetic field to generate heat-producing eddy currents in the object.

Infusion: Introduction of a fluid other than blood into a vein (e.g. a saline solution drip).

Inhalant: A substance that can be vaporized by mechanical means or by heat and carried into the respiratory tract by inhalation.

Intravenous: Administration of a drug by injection directly into a vein.

Ion: A charged atom or group of atoms formed by the dissociation of a molecule, often in an aqueous medium.

IQ: Installation qualification. This is a review of the equipment that establishes that the equipment meets its design specifications, and was installed in accordance with the design specifications. A term used in validation.

IR: Infrared.

Isotonic: Solutions that have the same osmotic pressure. A more specific definition is a solution in which cells neither swell nor shrink.

Istonicity: The situation obtained when the colligative or osmotic properties of a pharmaceutical are matched with those of a biological site of administration, frequently mucous membranes.

IV: Intravenous.

Kaolin: A family of clays containing combinations of hydrated alumina and silica.

Keratolytic: A medication used to treat conditions that lead to horny skin growths.

Kpsi: 1000 psi.

Latex: The milky juice of exudation of plants obtained by tapping the trunk (e.g. the fluid from a rubber plant).

LDPE: Low-density polyethylene.

Light-resistant container: A container that protects the contents from the effects of light.

Lipophilic: Having a strong affinity for oily or fatty substances.

LLDPE: Linear low-density polyethylene.

Lot or lot number: A lot refers to all the products made during a single run or manufacturing sequence on a piece of equipment or a complete production line. A run may last for a given quantity, for hours, or days, it normally denotes all products made in one sequence of starting and stopping the equipment when all raw materials are consumed or a given quantity is produced. A lot number is the assigned designation of that specific manufacturing sequence.

Lyophilization: Freeze-drying. The removal of water or solvent from a substance by applying a vacuum to the substance after it has been frozen.

Magma: Highly thickened suspensions for oral administration.

Mandrel: A metal rod or bar used as a core around which metal, glass, etc. is cast molded or shaped.

mg: Milligram.

Microbial control: Assembly of products in a controlled clean environment, followed by exposure to gamma radiation. This process reduces bioburder load but does not support a "sterile" label claim.

Microencapsulation: The encasement of small particles, either solid or liquid, within a shell that prevents their escape until the shell is ruptured by an external force or dissolved by a solvent.

Micron: One ten-thousandth of a centimeter.

Microorganisms, microbes: Living microscopic entities including bacteria and molds.

Multiple-dose container: A multiple-unit container for parenteral or ophthalmic formulations.

Multiple-unit container: One that permits the withdrawal of part of the contents while containing and protecting the un-withdrawn balance.

NDA: New Drug Application (FDA). Submission of all information necessary for review by the agency prior to approval of a new drug.

NDC: National Drug Code.

NF: National Formulary.

NWDA: The National Wholesale Druggists Association.

OFAS: Office of Food Additive Safety.

Offset: The process of using an intermediate cylinder to transfer an image from the image center to the substrate.

Ointment: A medicated preparation with the oleaginous base. More generally, a semisolid preparation intended for topical administration.

Oleaginous base: A base with the nature or quality of an oil.

ONPLDS: Office of Nutritional Products, Labeling, and Dietary Supplements.

Ophthalmic: Related to the eye.

OPP: Oriented polypropylene.

OTC: Over-the-counter.

Otic: Related to the ear.

Oxidation: Reaction with oxygen, more generally removal of electrons from an atom or molecule.

Parenteral: Introduction of substances into an organism by subcutaneous, intramuscular, intravenous, or intramedullary injection. Introduction by some other means than through the gastrointestinal tract.

pH: A measure of the hydrogen ion concentration in and the acidity of an aqueous solution.

Pharmaceutical: A manufactured, processed, or compounded form of a drug.

PIM: Product information management.

Plasticizer: A substance mixed into a plastic to decrease its stiffness and increase its softness.

Polymer: A high molecular weight molecule formed by reacting small molecules (monomers) together to form a long chain consisting of many monomer units.

Polyolefin: Any polymer whose monomer units are unsaturated hydrocarbons (olefins) containing only carbon and hydrogen. Polyethylene and polypropylene are the most common polyolefins used in packaging.

PPB: Parts per billion.

Prophylaxis: Prevention of disease or its spread by the administration of drugs and/or procedures.

Protocol: A set of procedures. Test or validation protocols are the set of instructions that govern how a test is run and how the data is to be reported.

PTFE: Polytetrafluoroethylene.

PVC: Polyvinyl chloride.

PVDC: Polyvinylidene chloride.

Pyrogen: Agent that causes a rise in body temperature, especially if injected. The most important pyrogen in sterile drug manufacture is endotoxins, a residue from gram-negative bacteria.

Resin: The term for a polymer in the form of small pellets that is packaged in a bag or in bulk and shipped to a processor. Sometimes a direct reference to the polymer itself.

Reverse osmosis: The process in which the solute in a solution is removed by forcing the solvent, against the normal osmotic pressure to flow through a membrane that is not permeable to the solute. Used to remove salts from seawater.

RH: Relative humidity.

Saturated: When used to describe a type of chemical bond or molecule, the bonding is saturated if no double or triple bonds exist, i.e. each atom is joined within the molecule to other atoms only by single bonds.

Scabacide: A substance that destroys the organism causing scabies.

Secondary package: The package that contains the primary package. It is not in direct contact with the product. Usually a box or carton.

Semipermeable-membrane: A membrane that permits the passage of one or more components of a solution but does not allow the passage of other components. Such membranes are usually permeable only by the solvent.

Shelf life: The time required for the potency of a drug to drop to 90% of its labeled potency.

Single-dose container: A single-unit container for primarily used for parenterals but also for other dosage forms that contains only one dose of product.

Single-unit container: A container that holds the quantity of drug intended for administration as a single dose promptly after the container is opened.

Sol: A colloidal solution or liquid phase of a colloidal solution.

Sterile: The absence of microorganisms.

Sterility testing: Tests performed to determine whether viable microorganisms are present. Commonly, the test involves immersing a component or system or flushing a fluid pathway with sterile microbial growth medium, incubation of the medium under conditions favorable for microbial growth, and observation of turbidity or other indication of microbial growth after a suitable incubation period.

Sterilization: A validated process used to render a product free from viable microorganisms. It is generally accepted that a terminally sterilized unit purporting to be sterile attain a sterility assurance level of $10-6$, i.e. probability of less than or equal to one chance in 1 million that a viable microorganism is present in the sterilized unit. Lower SALs may be validated as sterile in some cases.

Steroid: Fat-soluble organic compounds such as sterols, bile acids, and sex hormones.

Stratum corneum: The outermost layer of skin

Strip package: A package made by enclosing an object to be packaged such as a tablet between two webs and then sealing the webs together so that the seal completely surrounds the object being packaged.

Subcutaneous: Beneath the skin.

Sublingual: Under the tongue.

Substrate: Refers to the primary structural material or the surface of the primary material that is applied to other materials designed to alter the characteristics or properties of the original material.

Suppository: The dosage form designed for insertion into the rectum.

Surfactant: Any substance, normally a soap or detergent, that forms a compatibilizing boundary layer between two liquids or a liquid and solid. This layer leads to the staple dispersion one phase in another.

Suspension: Solid particles dispersed in a liquid. If the suspension is stable, it will resist the normal gravitational separation into two phases.

Systemic: Administration of a drug so that it gains access to the circulatory system. Can also refer to the introduction of a drug to all parts of the body to treat only one location.

Tensile strength: The resistance of a specimen to breaking when stressed longitudinally.

Therapeutic: Relating to the treatment of disease.

Thermoplastic: Describes any substance that becomes more pliable as it is heated. In packaging and molding, it refers to a material that can be formed when hot but become rigid after cooling.

Thermoset: Plastics that become rigid when heated or subjected to energy that initiates a chemical reaction at reactive sites linking all the individual polymer strands together permanently.

Tight container: A term defined by the USP that describes a container that protects its contents from contamination by extraneous liquids, solids, or gases from physical loss of the drug and from efflorescence, deliquescence, or evaporating under ordinary or customary conditions of handling, shipment, storage, and distribution.

Tincture: A solution of a drug in alcohol.

Topical: Administration of a drug to the skin surface or the lining of body cavities. Its effectiveness is limited to the localized areas to which it is applied.

Toxin: A noxious or poisonous substance formed during the growth of certain microorganisms.

Toxoid: A toxin that has been treated, e.g. with formaldehyde to destroy its toxic property but retain its antigenicity, i.e. its capability of stimulating the production of antitoxin antibodies and thus engendering immunity.

Transdermal: Administration of drugs through the skin.

Type I glass: Glass composed largely of silica and boric oxide that is very low in water extractable impurities.

Type II glass: Glass containing larger amounts of water-soluble sodium and calcium oxides than type I glass. Soda-lime glass with no boron-containing materials present.

Type III glass: Glass containing even greater quantities of water-extractable oxides than type II glass. A different and lower grade of soda-lime glass.

Unit-dose container: A single-unit container for products for administration by other than parenteral means as a singe dose direct from the container.

Unsaturated: In chemistry, molecules that contain more than one bond between two atoms. In polymers, it is usually referring to double and triple bonds between carbon and another atom.

USP: United States Pharmacopoeia.

USP-NF: United States Pharmacopoeia and National Formulary.

UV: Ultraviolet.

Validation: Testing and establishing documented evidence that provides a high degree of assurance that a specific process, component, or piece of equipment will consistently produce a product meeting its predetermined specifications and quality attributes.

Vasoconstrictors: Drugs that reduce the flow of body fluids by constricting the ducts, tubes, and canals through which these fluids flow. Often referred to drugs that constrict the circulatory system.

Vasodilators: Drugs that increase the flow of body fluids by relaxing the muscles surrounding the ducts, tubes, and canals through which those fluids flow.

Wavelength: The distance between identical points in a wave pattern. A measure of the energy content of light, the shorter the wavelength the higher the energy level.

Well-closed container: A USP term. A container that protects its contents from extraneous solids and physical loss under the ordinary and customary conditions of handling, shipment, and distribution.

Appendices

APPENDIX I
List of some commonly used additives

ABSORBENTS

Bentonite

Kaolin

Magnesium carbonate

Magnesium oxide

Magnesium silicate

Silica (cab-o-sil, syloid, aerosil)

Starch

Tricalcium phosphate

ANTIADHESIVES

Colloidal silica

Corn starch

DL-Leucine

Magnesium stearate

Metallic stearates

Sodium lauryl sulfate

Talc

ANTIFOAMING AGENTS

Ariacel C

Atlas G 1706

Ethylene glycol fatty acid ester

(Emcol EC-50)

G.M.S.

Propylene glycol monostearate

Span 65

Span 85

ANTIOXIDANTS

Acetone

Ascorbic acid

Ascorbyl palmitate

Benzoin

Beta-naphthol

Butylated hydroxytoluene

Butylated hydroxyanisole

Citric acid

Cysteine hydrochloride

Maleic acid

Monoisopropylcitrate

Nor-dihydroguaiaretic acid

Phenyl alphanapthlamine

Propyl gallate

Pyrogallol

Pyrocatechol

Sodium bisulfite

Sodium formaldehyde sulfoxylate

Dilauryl thiodipropionate	Sodium metabisulfite
Distearylthiodipropionate	Sodium sulfite
Ethylgallate	Sodium thiosulfate
Gallic acid	Thioglycerol
Glycerin	Thiosolbitol
Guaiac resin	Thiourea
Hydroquinone	Thioglycollic acid
Isoascorbic acid	Alpha tocopherol
Lecithin	Trihydroxybutyrophenone

COLORS

1. Natural

Alizarin	Hesperidin
Anattenes	Indigo
Caramel	Quercetin
Beta-carotene	Riboflavin
Carbon black	Rubia tinctorum
Carmic acid	Rutin
Chlorophyll	Saffron
Cochineal	Titanium dioxide
Curcumin	Turmeric
Ferric oxides (red and yellow)	Tyrian purple

2. Synthetic

Alizarin cyanine	Indigo carmine 73015
Amaranth I N 16785	Napthol blue black 20470
Brilliant Blue FCS 42090	Orange G 16 30
Carmoisine 14720	Ponceaux 4 16255
Eosine G 45380	Quinazarine 61565
Erythorosin 45430	Quinoline yellow SS 47000
Fast red E 16045	Resoroin brown 20170
Fast green FCF 42053	Sudan III 26100
Green S 44090	Sunset yello FCF 15185
Freen F 61570	Tartrazine 19140

EMULSIFYING AGENTS

1. Surfactants forming monomolecular films

Alkylpolyoxyethylene sulfates	Polyoxyethylene monolaurate (Atlas G 2127)
Benzalkonium chloride	(Polyoxyethylene alkylphenol (lgepal CA 630)

Cetrimide	Polyoxyethylene sorbitan monolaurate (Tween 20)
Dioctylsodium sulfosuccinate	Polyoxyethylene sorbitan mono-palmitate (Tween 40)
Lauryldimethylbenzylam-monium chloride	Polyoxyethylene sorbitan (Tween 80)
Lecithin	Polyoxyethylene laurylether (Brij 35)
N-cetyl N-ethyl mor-pholinium ethosulfate (Atlas G-263)	Monostearate (Myrj 52)
PEG 400 monostearate	Castor oil (Atlas G 1974)
Polyoxyethylene laurylether (Brij 30)	Potassium oleate
Polyoxyethylene mono-stearate (Myrj 45)	Sodium oleate
Propylene glycol mono-stearate	Sodium lauryl sulfate
Propylene glycol mono-stearate (Atlas G 917)	Sorbitan monopalmitate (Span 40)
Sorbitan monolaurate (Span 20)	Sorbitan monostearate (Arlacel 60)
Glyceryl monostearate (GMS)	Sodium laurate
Sorbitan sesquioleate (Alacel C)	Triethanolmine oleate
Potassium stearate	Triethanolamine stearate

2. Surfactants forming multimolecular films

Acacia	Hectorite
Agar	Magnesium hydroxide
Alginates	Pectin
Atapulgite	Silica gel
Bentonite	Tragacanth
Gelatin	Veegum

FLAVORING AGENTS

Almond	Oil of anise
Amyl acetate	Oil of bergamot
Anethol	Oil of caraway
Apricot	Oil of cardamom
Apple	Oil of cinnamon
Banana	Oil of clove

Benzaldehyde	Oil of coriander
Black currant	Oil of fennel
Blueberry	Oil of lemon
Butterscotch	Oil of lavender
Burgundy	Oil of nutmeg
Cherry	Oil of orange
Chocolate	Oil of narcissus
Custard	Oil of peppermint
Ethyl acetate	Oil of rosemary
Ethyl vanillin	Oil of rose
Eucalyptol	Oil of spearmint
Eugenol	Oil of thyme
Ginger	Orris root
Hyacinth	Peach
Jasmine	Phenyl ethyl alcohol
Lemongrass	Pineapple
Liquorice	Plum
Mango	Raspberry
Maple	Sandalwood
Methyl salicylate	Saffron
Melon	Strawberry
Narcissus	Thymol
Neroli	Vanillin
Violet	

FLOCCULATING AGENTS

Electrolytes like KH_2PO_4 $AlCl_3$, NaCl, etc.	Ionic and non-ionic surfactants hydrocolloids

PRESERVATIVES

Banzalkonium chloride	Boric acid and propyl alcohol
Benzoic acid and benzoates	Cetrimide
Benzylalcohol	Dichlorophene
Cetylpyridinium chloride	Ortho- and parachlorbenzoic acid
Chlorbutanol	Parahydroxybenzoates
Chlorothymol	Parachlor metacresol
p-Chlorphenylglyceryl ether	Parachlor metaxylenol
Dichlorometasylenol	p-Chlor phenylpropanediol
Dehydroacetic acid of phyenylmercuric acid	Phenyl mercuric nitrate and other salts

Formic acid	Phenol
Formaldehyde	Phenol hexachlorophene

SOLUBILIZING AGENTS

Atlas G 1690	PEG 400 monostearate
Atlas G 1794	Sodium oleate
Brij 35	Triethanolamine oleate
Igepal CA 630	Tween 20
Myrj 45	Tween 40
Myrj 49	Tween 60
Myrj 51	Tween 80
Myrj 52	

SUSPENDING AGENTS

Acacia	Hectorite
Agar	Hydroxyethyl cellulose
Alginates	Hydroxyl propyl cellulose
Attapulgite	Methyl celluloses
Bentonite	Microcrystalline cellulose
Carboxymethylcelluloses	Polyvinyl alcohol
Carbopol	Povidone
Carbomer	Psyllium seed gum
Cellulose poweder	Pectin
Chondrus	Tragacanth
Gelatin	Veegum
Guar gum	

SWEETENING AGENTS

Aspartyl phenylalanie	Maltose
Cyclamates	Mannitol
Dextrose	Neohesperidin dihydrochalcone
Fructose	Saccharin
Glycerin	Sorbitol
Glycyrrhizin	Sucrose
Honey	Xylitol
Lactose	

WETTING AGENTS

Tween 20	Span 20
Brij 30	Span 40

APPENDIX II
Units and conversion factors

Length	1 inch	= 0.0254 m
	1 ft	= 0.3048 m
Area	1 ft^2	= 0.0929 m^2
Volume	1 ft^3	= 0.0283 m^3
	1 gal Imp	= 0.004546 m^3
	1 gal US	= 0.003785 m^3 = 3.785 litres
	1 litre	= 0.001 m^3
Mass	1 lb	= 0.4536 kg
	1 mole	molecular weight in kg
Density	1 lb/ft^3	= 16.03 kg m^{-3}
Velocity	1 ft/sec	= 0.3048 m s^{-1}
Pressure	1 lb/m^2	= 6894 Pa
	1 torr	= 133.3 Pa
	1 atm	= 1.013 × 10^5 Pa = 760 mm Hg
	1 Pa	= 1 N m^{-2} = 1 kg m^{-1} s^{-2}
Force	1 Newton 1 lb ft s^{-2}	= 1 kg m s^{-2} = 1.49 kg m s^{-2}
Viscosity	1 cP	= 0.001 N s m^{-2} = 0.001 Pa s
	1 lb/ft sec	= 1.49 N s m^{-2} = 1.49 kg m^{-1} s^{-2}
Energy	1 Btu	= 1055 J
	1 cal	= 4.186 J
Power	1 kW1 W	= 1 kJ s^{-1} = 1 J s^{-1}
	1 horsepower	= 745.7 W = 745.7 J s^{-1} = 0.746 kW
	1 ton refrigeration	= 3.519 kW
Temperature units	(°F)	= 5/9 (°C) = 5/9 (K)
Heat-transfer coefficient	1 Btu ft^{-2} h^{-1} °F^{-1}	= 5.678 J m^{-2} s^{-1}°C
Thermal conductivity	1 Btu ft^{-1} h^{-1} °F^{-1}	= 1.731 J m^{-1} s^{-1}°C^{-1}
Constants	Π	3.1416
	e (base of natural logs)	2.7183
	R	8.314 kJ mole^{-1} K^{-1} or 0.08206 m^3 atm mole^{-1} K^{-1}

(M) Mega = 10^6, (k) kilo = 10^3, (H) hecto = 10^2, (m) milli = 10^{-3}, (μ) micro = 10^{-6}

APPENDIX III
Standard sieves

S. No.	Aperture $(m \times 10^{-3})$	ISO nominal aperture $(m \times 10^{-3})$	US no.	Tyler no.
1.	22.6		7/8 in.	0.883 in.
2.	16.0	16	5/8 in.	0.624 in.
3.	11.2	11.2	7/16 in.	0.441 in.
4.	8.0	8.00	5/16 in.	2 1/2 mesh
5.	5.66	5.66	No. 3 1/2	3 1/2 mesh
6.	4.00	4.00	5	5 mesh
7.	2.83	2.80	7	7 mesh
8.	2.00	2.00	10	9 mesh
9.	1.41	1.41	14	12 mesh
10.	1.00	1.00	18	16 mesh
11.	0.71	0.710	25	24 mesh
12.	0.500	0.500	35	32 mesh
13.	0.354	0.355	45	42 mesh
14.	0.250	0.250	60	60 mesh
15.	0.177	0.180	80	80 mesh
16.	0.125	0.125	120	115 mesh
17.	0.088	0.090	170	170 mesh
18.	0.063	0.063	230	250 mesh
19.	0.044	0.045	325	325 mesh

*Note: $0.50 \, m \times 10^{-3}$ aperture = 35 US No. = 32 mesh

Index